Learn to Cook
Asian Cooking for Health

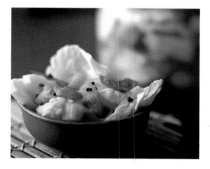

Asian cooking is not only healthy but also flavorful. This handy book contains over 40 nutritious and delicious recipes—like Chicken and Ginseng Soup, Fresh Tofu Salad and Fish Soup with Fennel.

PERIPLUS

Contents

MAIL ORDER SOURCES

Finding the ingredients for Asian home cooking has become very simple. Most super-markets carry staples such as soy sauce, fresh ginger, and fresh lemongrass. Almost every large metropolitan area has Asian markets serving the local population—just check your local business directory. With the Internet, exotic Asian ingredients and cooking utensils can be easily found online. The following list is a good starting point of online merchants offering a wide variety of goods and services.

http://www.asiafoods.com

http://www.geocities.com/MadisonAvenue/8074/VarorE.html

http://dmoz.org/Shopping/Food/Ethnic_and_Regional/Asian/

http://templeofthai.com/

http://www.orientalpantry.com/

http://www.zestyfoods.com/

http://www.thaigrocer.com/Merchant/index.htm

http://asianwok.com/

http://www.indiangrocerynet.com/

http://www.orientalfoodexpress.com/

http://www.i-clipse.com/ (Pacific Rim Gourmet)

http://www..ethnicfoodsco.com/ShoppingAndMoreMain.html

http://www.thecmccompany.com/

http://www.ethnicgrocer.com/

Who hasn't benefited from a bowl of chicken soup when they've been sick with a cold or flu? That warm and soothing bowl of soup is more than just comfort food. Chicken soup does help clear nasal clog. Not only do the vapors from the hot liquid clear stuffy nasal passages, but the onions and garlic used in the soup also have antiseptic qualities.

People have known about the health-promoting and healing qualities of various foods almost as long as there have been people, but Asian cooks have made an art of cooking for health. Indeed, much of what you see on the shelves in Asian food shops is also available in herbal remedies from the Chinese doctor around the corner.

This book is a collection of recipes that not only taste fabulous, but can help you and your family maintain optimum health. Many of the ingredients in these recipes are more than just nutritious—from the everyday onion and garlic to Chinese red dates and ginseng, they have actual medicinal value. In addition to having loads of vitamin C, the dates are said to improve blood quality and cure insomnia. Ginseng has so many healing properties that part of its scientific name is panax, as in panacea. This general tonic is used for nearly everything from enhancing athletic performance to soothing motion sickness.

The tiger lily buds, bamboo pith and wolfberries in the wonderfully named "Forget Your Troubles Soup" are said to calm "liver fire" and thus relax the nervous system. Ginger, used often in the West to settle stomachs, has a long list of benefits, reportedly including curing chills in elephants! And that protein-rich culinary chameleon tofu has no cholesterol and minimal saturated fats, but heaps of isoflavones and phytoestrogens.

So experiment with some of these exotic but easy-to-find ingredients. You'll be surprised how tasty keeping healthy can be.

Basic Asian Ingredients

Aromatic ginger, also known as *kencur* or *cekor*, is sometimes mistakenly called lesser galangal. This ginger-like root with a unique, camphor-like flavor should be used sparingly. Wash it and scrape off the skin before using. Dried sliced *kencur* powder can be used as a substitute. Soak dried slices in boiling water for approximately 30 minutes; use $1/2$–1 teaspoon of powder for 1 in ($2^1/_2$ cm) of fresh root.

Bamboo shoots are used fresh, dried or canned in Asian cookery. Fresh shoots are sweet and crunchy. Peel, slice and boil them for about 30 minutes before adding to dishes. Soak and boil dried shoots before use. Drain and boil canned bamboo shoots in fresh water for 5 minutes to remove the metallic taste.

Basil of many varieties is used in Asian cooking. **Thai basil** (*krapow* or *kaprao*), also known as Asian basil, has pungent leaves on purple stems and imparts a heady and minty flavor and aroma to dishes. **Lemon basil** (*kemangi*) has smaller, slightly hairy leaves and a lemony aroma and flavor. In general, Italian basil or fresh cilantro (coriander leaves) can be substituted in cooked dishes and fresh mint or basil in uncooked ones.

Bonito flakes are the shavings of dried, smoked and cured bonito fish, sold in fine or coarse flakes in small plastic packs. Fine flakes are used as a garnish, while coarse flakes are used to make bonito fish stock (**dashi**). Store unused portions in an airtight container or plastic bag.

Chilies come in many shapes and sizes. The relatively mild large red or green chilies are commonly used, while the tiny bird's-eye chilies provide much more heat. **Dried red chilies** are sometimes preferred for the brighter color they give to cooked dishes, and for their smoky aroma. **Chili oil**, cooking oil that has been infused with chilies, is also used in some dishes.

Chinese red dates, also known as jujubes, are the olive-shaped, dark red fruit of a small thorny evergreen tree. Red dates have a slightly astringent, prune-like flavor and are available dried at Asian food shops.

Daikon is a variety of large white radish and is also known as Japanese or Asian radish. They are milder than small red radishes, more like a white carrot actually. Daikon can be eaten raw in salads, pickled, or used in stir-fries, soups and stews. It has a sweet and zesty flavor with a mild bite.

Dashi powder is used to make *dashi* fish stock and as a basic seasoning in many Japanese recipes including soups and salad dressings. It may be substituted with soup stock powder or bouillon cubes.

Dried shrimp are a popular seasoning in many Asian dishes. Choose dried shrimps that are pink in color and soak in water to soften before use. Look for brightly colored, plump dried shrimp. Soak for about 5 minutes to soften before using.

Dried shrimp paste, also called *belachan*, is an extremely pungent paste made from fermented shrimp. It is available in jars or firm brown blocks. Unless it is going to be fried as part of a spice paste, it needs to be toasted before cooking. Either wrap it in foil and roast or dry-fry it in a pan, or toast it above a gas flame on the back of a spoon.

Fish sauce, a fermented fish product called *nam pla* in Thai and *nuoc mam* in Vietnamese, is a basic seasoning ingredient throughout Southeast Asia.

Galangal, which is known as *lengkuas* in Singapore and Malaysia, is a member of the ginger family. This aromatic root, which resembles pink-colored ginger imparts a distinctive flavor to many dishes prepared throughout Southeast Asia. It is available fresh or bottled in brine (often more tender than fresh) in Asian food shops and well-stocked supermarkets. The fresh root can be sliced and frozen for future use. If the root is tough, steam it over boiling water for about 10–15 minutes before chopping and processing it.

Ghee is the rich clarified butter oil used as the main oil in Indian cooking. It is made from cow or water buffalo milk by removing the milk solids from the oil. If ghee is not available, substitute with vegetable oil or butter.

Japanese rice is a short-grain variety that is slightly more starchy than Thai or Chinese long-grain rice. It is available at Asian food shops and most supermarkets. It may be substituted with any short- or medium-grain rice.

Japanese seven-spice chili powder or *shichimi-togarashi* blends chili pepper with other ingredients including sansho and nori flakes. The mixtures are sprinkled over various dishes including soups.

Kaffir lime leaves are dark green leaves shaped like a figure of eight. They add an intense fragrance to dishes and are used whole in soups and curries, or shredded finely and added to salads. Kaffir leaves may be substituted with regular lime leaves, lemon leaves or lime zest.

Lemongrass is an aromatic stalk that gives a delectable lemon flavor and fragrance to any dish. The stems are tough and need cutting into useable lengths with a sharp knife. The tender inner part of the base is ground to a paste, or the whole stem bruised and used to flavor curries and sauces.

Long beans, sometimes called yard-long beans or snake beans, taste and look like green beans. They grow up to 3 ft (1 m) in length, although they are usually picked when about 18 in (50 cm) long.

Mirin is a sweet liquid made by mixing and fermenting steamed glutinous rice with *shoju* (a distilled spirit similar to vodka). It adds a lovely glaze to grilled foods and is used to flavor soup stocks, marinades and dressings.

Miso is a fermented paste made from soybeans and/or wheat. **Red miso paste** is red to brown in color, high in protein and tastes more salty than **white miso paste**, which is sweeter and milder than red miso. Miso is used to enhance the flavor of soups, stocks and dressings, and as a grilling baste for meat and fish. Miso loses its flavor and digestive properties if allowed to boil. Refrigerate after opening.

Mushrooms and fungi of various types, fresh and dried, are used in Asian cooking. **Shiitake mushrooms**, also known as **Chinese black mushrooms**, are large and meaty, and used in soups, stir-fries and side dishes, or as a meat substitute. **Straw mushrooms** add a smooth texture to dishes and they are very high in protein. Fresh straw mushrooms can be found in specialty produce markets, but they are more readily available canned.

Noodles come in many varieties, both fresh and dried, and are normally made from rice, wheat or beans. **Bean thread vermicelli** (*tang fen* or *tang hoon*), also called cellophane noodles, are thin translucent threads made from the starch of green mung beans. The dried noodles must be soaked briefly in hot water before using. **Egg noodles** are generally made from wheat and egg and are available in round or flat shapes in a variety of sizes. **Rice vermicelli** are made from rice flour, and are dried noodles that can be easily rehydrated by soaking in hot water for a few minutes, then rinsing before further boiling or frying. **Rice stick noodles** are similar to rice vermicelli except that they are flatter and larger, ranging in width from very narrow to about $1/3$ in (8 mm). **Soba noodles** are slender Japanese noodles made from buckwheat.

Palm sugar is made from the sap of palm trees and ranges in color from golden brown to dark brown. It is less sweet than white sugar, and has a distinctive, maple syrup-like flavor. If palm sugar is not available, substitute with dark brown sugar, maple sugar or maple syrup.

Pickled ginger is thinly sliced young ginger roots that are pickled in a brine of rice vinegar and sugar. *Shoga* is red or salmon pink, and *gari* is pale yellow. It adds the crisp flavor of ginger to fish and vegetable dishes and is a tangy addition to stir-fried dishes.

Preserved Chinese vegetable (*tang chye* or *tung choi*) is salted or pickled mustard greens. It is available in jars in Asian food shops.

Rice wine is used in Asian cooking as a tenderizer and flavoring. A good alternative to rice wine is dry sherry or sake.

Sake is a brewed alcoholic beverage also known as Japanese rice wine. Chinese rice wine or dry sherry may be used as a substitute.

Sansho pepper, closely related to the Sichuan pepper, is a mildly hot Japanese seasoning made from the berries of the prickly ash tree, which are dried and ground into a powder.

Seaweeds of various types are used in Asian cooking. **Nori** is a type of seaweed that has been pressed into very thin sheets and baked until it is dry and crisp. Before use, hold a nori sheet over an open flame for a few seconds so that it becomes lightly toasted, or toast it in a toaster oven. **Wakame** is a green ribbon-like member of the brown algae family. Seaweeds of various types are available in Asian food shops and many health food shops.

Sesame oil is extracted from sesame seeds that have been well toasted, producing a dark, dense, aromatic oil with a nutty, smoky flavor. It is often used in marinades, sauces and soups, or as a table condiment. The most common variety is Chinese sesame oil. **Japanese sesame oil** is much less concentrated and can be substituted with a mixture of approximately two parts Chinese sesame oil to one part cooking oil.

Sesame paste is made from ground, roasted sesame seeds and comes in glass jars containing oil. It is quite hard and needs to be mixed with a little sesame oil or water to make it into a smooth paste. If you can't find it, use Middle Eastern tahini mixed with sesame oil to give it a more pronounced flavor.

Shiso leaves are flat green leaves with a flavor similar to spearmint, basil and mint. Fresh basil, or a mix of fresh basil and spearmint are the closest substitutes.

Sichuan pepper, also known as flower pepper, is one of the ingredients in five-spice powder. Sichuan peppercorns are available both whole and ground. **Sichuan pepper-salt powder** is made by dry-roasting 2 tablespoons salt, 1 table-spoon Sichuan peppercorns and 1 tea-spoon white peppercorns until fragrant and just beginning to smoke, then grind-ing the mixture to a powder in a spice grinder or with a mortar and pestle.

Soy sauce, brewed from wheat, salt and soy beans, is available in several forms. The most common is **regular light soy sauce**, a clear medium brown liquid with a salty taste, often used as a table condi-ment. **Dark soy sauce** (Chinese brands are often labelled "superior soy sauce") is dense black and thicker, less salty and with a malty tang. **Black sweet soy sauce** receives additional richness from extend-ed fermentation and is reduced to con-centrate the flavor. A touch of molasses is also added. **Sweet soy sauce** (*kecap manis*) is a very thick sweetened variety found mainly in Indonesia. It is well worth spending a little extra to purchase high-quality soy sauce of any type.

Tamarind is widely available dried in pulp form. To use, soak the specified quantity of pulp in water for five min-utes. Squeeze the pulp with your fingers, then stir and strain the mixture to remove the solids. Discard the solids and use the tamarind juice.

Tiger lily buds (golden needles) are the unopened buds of a variety of Chinese day lily and are prized for their earthy flavor. The buds are available dried at Asian food shops, and are soaked and their tough stems removed before use.

Tofu, also know as beancurd, is made of soybeans in a process that is much like making cheese. This protein-rich product has little flavor on its own, but readily absorbs the flavors of whatever sauces it is cooked in. Cakes of fresh tofu are available in many consistencies, including **soft**, **medium**, **firm**, **extra firm** and the creamy **silken**. Fresh tofu is usually sold in cakes in sealed plastic tubs of water. Once opened, store tofu in the refrigera-tor in a sealed container with enough fresh water to cover it. Tofu is also avail-able in many other forms including **dried tofu**, which is dehydrated tofu sold in packages of little cakes about 2 in (5 cm) square and $1/2$ in (1 cm) thick.

Turmeric, when fresh, resembles ginger until its bright yellow interior is exposed. It has an aromatic and spicy fragrance, when fresh. In its dried and ground form, it is a basic ingredient of curry powders. The color of ground turmeric tends to fade if stored too long.

Wasabi, or Japanese horseradish, is a pungent root. It tastes similar to ginger and hot mustard. It is sold fresh, as a pre-pared paste, or in dried powdered form.

Water spinach (*kangkong*) is a nutritious leafy green vegetable also known as water convolvulus. Young shoots may be eaten raw as part of a salad platter or with a dip. The leaves and tender stems are usu-ally braised. This leafy vegetable does not keep well, but can be refrigerated.

Sichuan Pickled Cabbage (China)

Pickled cabbage dishes, such as the famous *kimchees* of Korea, are traditional fare throughout Asia, and even Europe has its versions, like the German *sauerkraut*. Pickled cabbage has a wide range of benefits to human health. It contains live enzymes that facilitate digestion of other foods that are eaten with it and it reduces cholesterol. According to Chinese medicine it tones the spleen and stomach, and the chilies, Sichuan peppercorns and other spices in the Sichuan version drive dampness from the body and protect it from parasites and microbes. This dish can be prepared in large quantities and kept in a covered jar in the refrigerator so that you can serve a small side dish of it with your all main meals.

12 cups (3 liters) water
1 large or 2 small heads of ordinary round white cabbage, washed and leaves separated (tear leaves in chunks)
6 slices ginger
1 large leek (about 8 oz/ 225 g), halved lengthwise then cut in 2-in (5-cm) lengths
2 fresh red chilies, halved lengthwise then cut in three
4 stalks fresh celery, cut into 2-in (5-cm) slices
1 medium carrot, cut on an angle into 3/4-in (2-cm) slices
1 medium daikon (about 7 oz/200 g), cut on an angle into 3/4-in (2-cm) slices

Seasonings
10 Sichuan peppercorns
3 cups (750 ml) high proof vodka
2 teaspoons salt (preferably sea salt)

1 Pour the water into a clean wide-mouthed glass or ceramic vessel that will hold at least 16 cups (4 liters).
2 Add the Seasonings, then the cabbage, then all the remaining ingredients on top of the cabbage. Do not stir. Cover the vessel tightly with a lid (place a weight on top if necessary to keep a tight seal), and set aside to pickle for 3 days.
3 After 3 days, taste to see if it has fermented sufficiently (this depends on climate and season). If ready, serve small dishes of the vegetables with any meal. After 5 days, you should keep the pickled cabbage in the refrigerator, where it will keep for another 7–10 days.

This is the basic Sichuan method of preparing pickled cabbage. If you know other ways, such as for Korean kimchee, you may freely mix the various methods to come up with your own favorite combinations. Serving this dish with a meal is particularly beneficial to digestion when there are a lot of meat, poultry and seafood dishes on the table.

Serves 4
Preparation time: 15 mins
Pickling time: 3–5 days

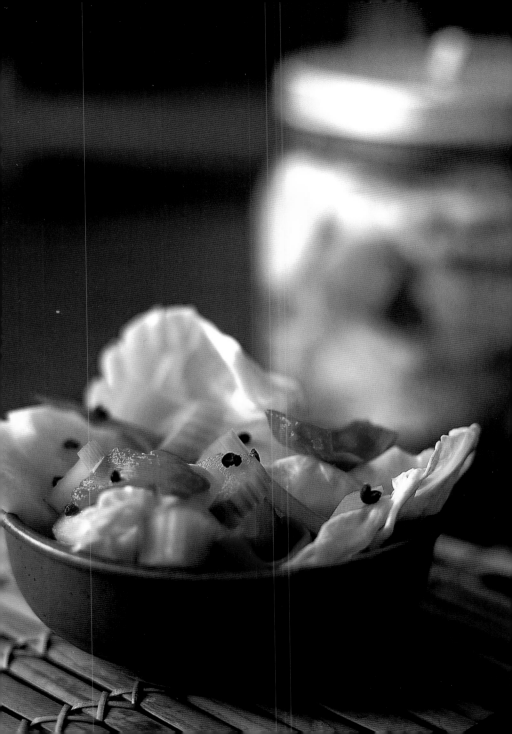

Pickled Beansprouts and Carrots (China)

12 oz (4$^1/_2$ cups/350 g) fresh beansprouts
2 scallions, cut into 2-in (5-cm) lengths
1 carrot, peeled and coarsely grated
1 tablespoon salt
$^3/_4$ cup (185 ml) white vinegar
2 tablespoons sugar
1 cup (250 ml) water

1 Combine the beansprouts, scallions and carrot in a large mixing bowl and set aside.
2 Combine the salt, vinegar, sugar and water in a saucepan and bring to the boil over medium heat, stirring until the sugar and salt dissolve. Remove from the heat and set aside to cool.
3 Combine the vinegar mixture with the vegetables in a mixing bowl and marinate for at least 1 hour. Drain before serving.

Serves 4–6
Preparation time: **10 mins**
Cooking time: **10 mins + 1 hour standing**

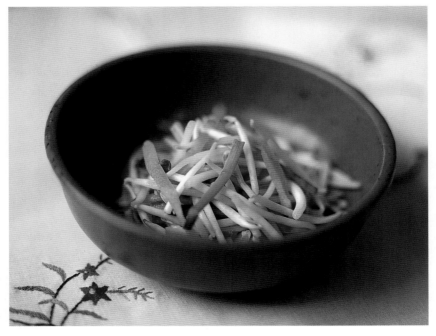

Pickled Chinese Cabbage (Japan)

1 head (about 13 oz/
375 g) Chinese Napa
cabbage
1 tablespoon salt
3 teaspoons sugar
1 red chili, seeded and
thinly sliced (optional)

Serves 8–10
Preparation time: 5–8 mins
+ overnight standing

1 Remove the core of the cabbage, making sure the
cabbage remains in one piece. Wash well, shake to
remove excess water and squeeze as much liquid from
the cabbage as possible. Pat dry with paper towels.
Cut the cabbage into several $1^1/_4$-in (3-cm) sections
widthwise.
2 Rub half of the salt, sugar and chili into the sections
of cabbage. Sprinkle a little salt and sugar in the base
of a plastic bowl and stand each section of cabbage
upright, side by side. Top with the remaining salt,
sugar and chili, and place a heavy weight on top to
weigh the cabbage down. Cover the bowl and let
stand overnight in a cool place or in the refrigerator.
3 To serve, rinse the cabbage leaves well, then drain
and cut into bite-sized pieces and arrange on a plate or
in a shallow bowl.

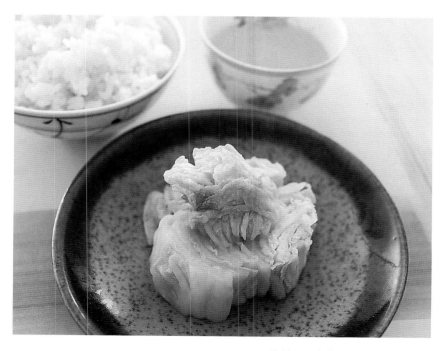

Cucumber and Daikon Salad (Japan)

1 lb (450 g) daikon, peeled and julienned (about 3 cups), soaked in cold water for 10 minutes and drained
2 baby cucumbers (about 8 oz/220 g), shaved into long, thin strips using a vegetable peeler, stopping before you reach the seeds (about $^2/_3$ cup)
1 small carrot, julienned (about $^2/_3$ cup)
$^1/_2$ small onion, thinly sliced (about $^1/_3$ cup), soaked in water and drained
2 sheets *nori*, lightly toasted, halved and cut into thin strips (see page 6)
2 teaspoons black sesame seeds

Dressing
2 tablespoons soy sauce
2 tablespoons *mirin*
1 teaspoon white sugar
2 tablespoons rice wine vinegar
$^1/_2$ teaspoon *dashi* powder dissolved in 1 tablespoon water

1 Combine all the Dressing ingredients in a small bowl and set aside.
2 To assemble the salad, toss the daikon, cucumbers, carrots and drained onion slices in a medium bowl. Pile the tossed vegetables high on a serving plate. Immediately before serving, pour over the prepared Dressing and top with roasted *nori* and sesame seeds.

Serves 4–6
Preparation time: **15 mins**

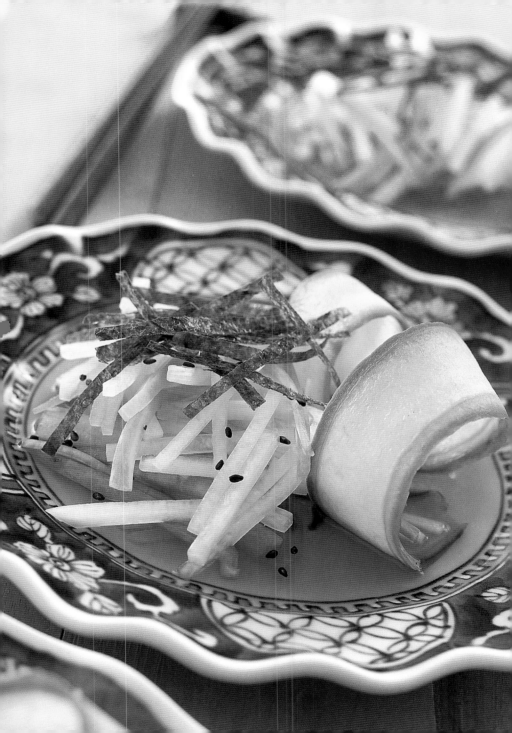

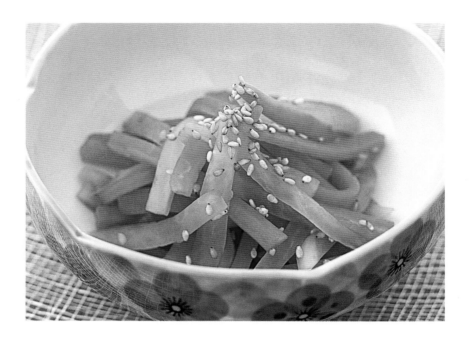

Daikon and Carrot Salad
with Roasted Sesame (Japan)

1³/₄ cups (440 ml) water
1 tablespoon salt
10 oz (300 g) daikon, julienned
¹/₂ medium carrot, julienned
3 tablespoons rice wine vinegar
1 tablespoon *mirin*
1 tablespoon soy sauce
1 tablespoon roasted sesame seeds

1 Place 1¹/₂ cups (375 ml) of the water and the salt in a medium bowl. Add the daikon and carrot and leave to soak for 30 minutes, then drain and set aside.
2 Combine the vinegar, remaining water (¹/₄ cup), *mirin* and soy sauce in a small saucepan. Add carrot and daikon and simmer. Remove from heat and set aside to cool.
3 When ready to serve, squeeze gently to remove excess vinegar mixture. Place vegetables in small bowls and serve sprinkled with sesame seeds.

Serves 4–6
Preparation time: 5 mins + 30 mins soaking
Cooking time: 5 mins

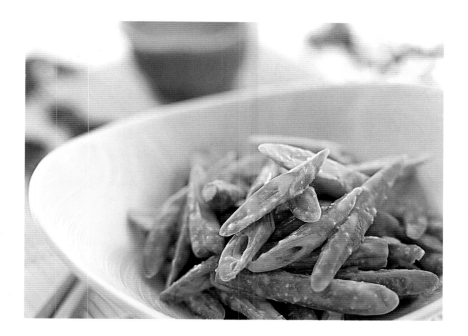

Green Beans in Sesame Dressing (Japan)

6 oz (170 g) fresh or
  frozen green beans
2 cups (500 ml) water
1 teaspoon salt
1 1/2 tablespoons sesame
  paste
1 teaspoon sugar
2 teaspoons soy sauce
1 tablespoon sake
1 teaspoon rice vinegar
1/4 teaspoon *dashi*
  powder dissolved in
  1 tablespoon water
1 teaspoon white miso

1 If using fresh beans, remove the tops and tails and cut beans into 2-in (5-cm) lengths. Bring the water and salt to the boil in a medium saucepan and blanch the beans until just tender and a bright green color, about 3–5 minutes. Immediately plunge into ice cold water until cold, then drain well.

2 Combine the sesame paste, sugar, soy sauce, sake, vinegar, *dashi* and miso in a large mixing bowl and toss beans through the mixture. Serve warm or at room temperature.

Serves 4
Preparation time: **10 mins**
Cooking time: **5 mins**

Spinach and Bean Thread Salad (China)

This is a classic Chinese *lengpan* (cold dish), in which briefly poached ingredients are tossed in a strongly seasoned sauce. A dish like this usually appears on the table first, to serve as a *kai wei* ("stomach opener", or appetizer) or as a *jiou tsai* ("wine food", or hors d'oeuvres). There are many variations of this dish, but the one given here is a tried-and-true favorite of the ages.

$^1/_2$ lb (225 g) fresh spinach, washed and drained
1 small package (3$^1/_2$ oz/ 100 g) dried bean thread vermicelli
2 tablespoons finely chopped garlic

Sauce
1 tablespoon soy sauce
1 teaspoon sesame oil
$^1/_2$ teaspoon vinegar
1 teaspoon sugar
$^1/_2$ teaspoon salt
$^1/_2$ teaspoon freshly ground black pepper
1 tablespoon *wasabi*

Serves 4
Preparation time: 10 mins
Cooking time: 5 mins

1 Bring a large pot of water to the boil, add the spinach and allow the water to return to the boil, about 2 minutes. Immediately remove the spinach to a colander and reserve the boiling water. Rinse under cool water and set aside to drain.
2 Mix all the Sauce ingredients and set aside.
3 Soak the dried bean threads in cool water for a few minutes, then squeeze them dry by hand, and drop them into the reserved boiling water. Simmer for 2–3 minutes, then drain and set aside (do not rinse in cool water).
4 Lightly squeeze the spinach to remove any excess water, then place on a cutting board and cut into 2-in (5-cm) pieces. Do the same with the bean threads.
5 Place the spinach and bean threads in a large bowl, add the garlic and the Sauce, and toss until the spinach and bean threads are well mixed and completely coated with the Sauce. Transfer to a serving dish and serve.

Adding some form of seaweed enhances the flavor and the nutritional value of this dish. If the seaweed requires cooking, poach it the same way you poached the spinach and bean threads, then cut it to a similar size. Some cooks like to garnish the finished dish with a sprinkling of chopped fresh scallions.

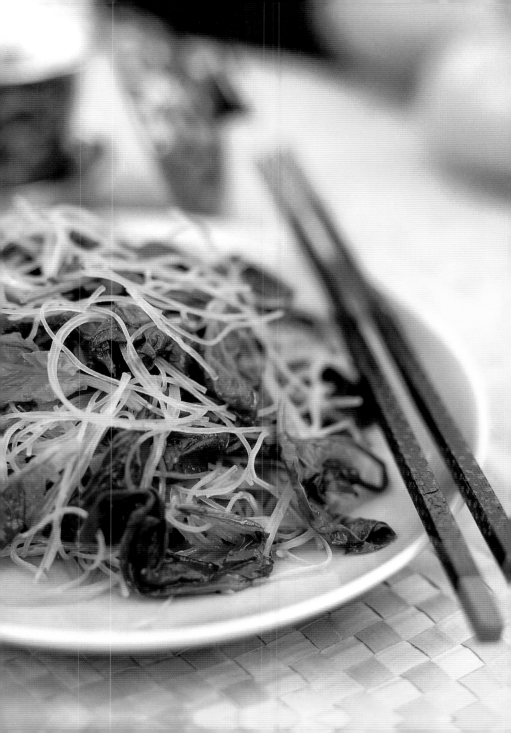

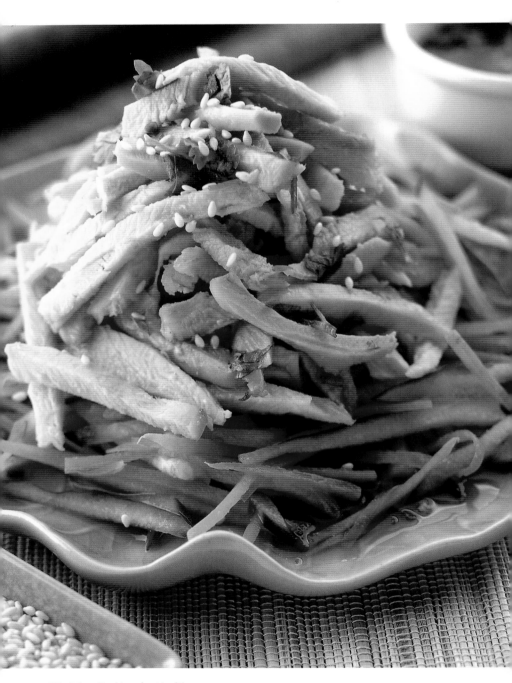

Chinese Chicken Salad (China)

10 oz (300 g) boneless chicken breast meat
2 small carrots (about 4 oz/120 g), julienned
1 small cucumber (about 5 oz/140 g), julienned
2 tablespoons toasted peanuts, coarsely chopped or toasted sesame seeds
2 scallions, thinly sliced
1 tablespoon coarsely chopped fresh cilantro (coriander leaves)
1 red chili, seeds removed and thinly sliced (optional)

Marinade
2 tablespoons ginger juice, pressed from freshly grated ginger
2 tablespoons rice wine
$^1/_3$ teaspoon salt
1 teaspoon sugar

Sauce
$^1/_4$ cup (60 ml) chicken stock (made from chicken bouillon cubes)
3 tablespoons oyster sauce
1 teaspoon sugar
$^1/_4$ teaspoon pepper
1 teaspoon sesame oil

1 Combine the Marinade ingredients in a mixing bowl, mix thoroughly then set aside.
2 Add the chicken to the Marinade, toss to coat thoroughly, then set aside to marinate for 1 hour.
3 When marinated, drain the chicken and place it in a steamer to cook for 10 minutes. Remove and set aside to cool, then cut or tear the meat into strips.
4 Arrange the carrot and cucumber on a platter and top with the chicken.
5 Put the Sauce ingredients into a small saucepan and bring to the boil. Spoon the hot Sauce over the chicken. Sprinkle with the chopped peanuts and the sliced scallions, cilantro and sliced chili, if using, and serve.

Serves 2
Preparation time: **40 mins**
Cooking time: **20 mins**

Mixed Vegetable Salad with Spicy Peanut Dressing (Indonesia)

8 oz (3 cups/225 g) water spinach or other green leafy vegetables, washed and drained
8 oz (3 cups/225 g) spinach leaves, washed and drained
8 oz (1 1/4 cups/225 g) long beans, sliced
8 oz (2 cups/225 g) bean-sprouts, tails removed, washed and drained
Few sprigs Thai basil
Deep-fried shrimp crackers, (optional)

Peanut Dressing
1–2 large red chilies, sliced
2–3 red bird's eye chilies (optional)
2 teaspoons finely chopped aromatic ginger or galangal
4 cloves garlic, dry roasted until brown, peeled
3 kaffir lime leaves, blanched in boiling water to soften, sliced
1/2 teaspoon dried shrimp paste, toasted (page 7)
1 tablespoon tamarind pulp soaked in 1/4 cup (60 ml) water (page 7)
2 teaspoons salt
1/2 cup (90 g) finely chopped palm sugar
1 1/2 cups (250 g) peanuts, dry roasted and skinned
2 cups (500 ml) hot water

1 To prepare the Peanut Dressing, process the chilies, aromatic ginger, garlic, lime leaves, shrimp paste, tamarind water, salt and palm sugar in a spice grinder or blender until smooth. Chop the peanuts coarsely in a food processor. Add the spice paste and pulse a few of times. Add the water and pulse to make a thick sauce.
2 Bring a large pot of water to the boil, add the water spinach and allow the water to return to the boil, about 2 minutes. Immediately remove the water spinach to a colander and reserve the boiling water. Rinse under cool water and set aside to drain again. Repeat this process separately with the spinach, beans and beansprouts. Drain each thoroughly and chop both lots of spinach coarsely.
3 Arrange the vegetables on a plate and either spoon the Peanut Dressing over the vegetables or serve it separately. Garnish with Thai basil and shrimp crackers, if using, and serve at room temperature.

*To prepare **dried shrimp crackers**, deep-fry in very hot oil. The oil is hot enough if a test cracker puffs up to three times its original size within one minute. Prepared shrimp crackers are also available in packets from Asian food stores.*
If using roasted salted peanuts, reduce the amount of salt in the Peanut Dressing to 1/2 teaspoon. If a milder dressing is desired, reduce the number of chilies used.

Serves 4
Preparation time: **30 mins**
Cooking time: **30–35 mins**

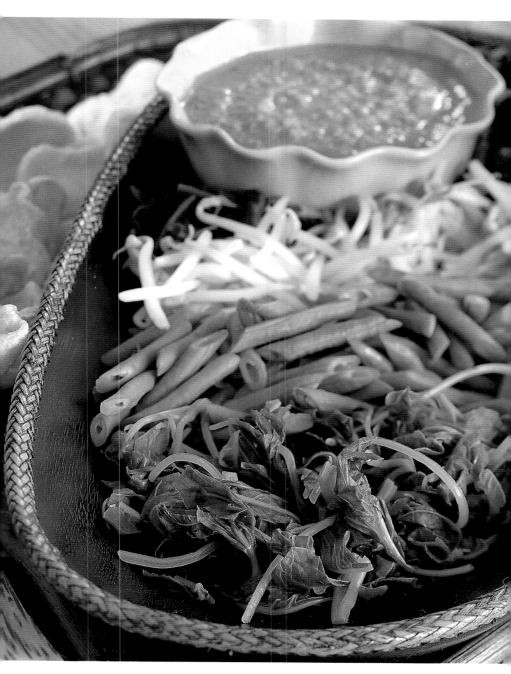

Cucumber Salad with Spicy Dressing (China)

1 lb (450 g) baby
cucumbers, washed
2 teaspoons salt
2 tablespoons finely
chopped garlic
2 fresh red chilies, cut at
an angle into thin slices

Dressing
1 tablespoon sugar
$1/_2$ teaspoon ground
Sichuan pepper
1 tablespoon apple cider
or other vinegar
2 teaspoons sesame oil
$1/_2$ teaspoon freshly
ground black pepper

1 Cut each cucumber in half lengthwise, then cut each half into $1^1/_4$ in (3 cm) sections widthwise. Place the cucumbers in a bowl, add the salt, toss to coat the pieces evenly, and let stand for 15 minutes. Rinse the cucumbers in cold water to remove the salt, then drain in a colander.
2 Meanwhile, combine the Dressing ingredients, mix well and set aside.
3 Place the drained cucumbers into a serving bowl and add the garlic, chili and Dressing. Stir to blend the flavors and serve.

Serves 4–6
Preparation time: **20 mins**
Assembling time: **2 mins**

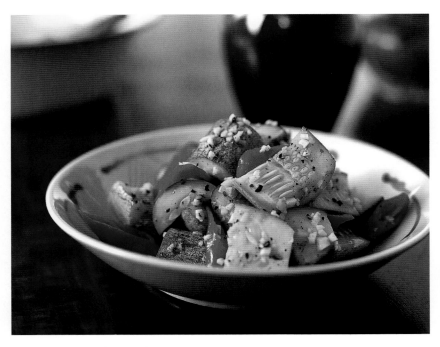

Green Papaya Salad (Thailand)

3 tablespoons lime juice
3 tablespoons fish sauce
1 tablespoon sugar
2 teaspoons chopped
  garlic
1 red or green chili,
  chopped
1 large tomato, cut into
  8 wedges
3 cups (600 g) coarsely
  grated green (unripe)
  papaya
1 carrot, coarsely grated
2 tablespoons coarsely
  chopped mint, plus
  extra leaves to garnish
2 tablespoons sesame
  seeds, toasted

1 To make the salad, combine all the ingredients in a large serving bowl and toss well to combine. Garnish with the reserved mint leaves and serve.

Cooked fresh shrimps or beef jerky may be added to this refreshing and unusual salad to turn it into a main dish.

Serves 3–4
Preparation time: **15 mins**

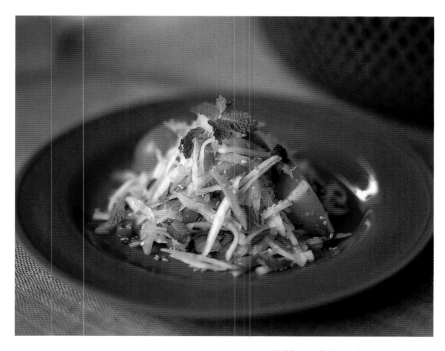

Braised Tofu with Mushrooms (China)

4 tablespoons olive oil

7 oz (200 g) firm tofu, cut into 1$^1/_2$-cm ($^3/_4$-in) thick slices

$^1/_4$ teaspoon salt

1 clove garlic, sliced

1 teaspoon grated ginger

10 fresh Chinese or shiitake mushrooms, whole or halved

1 medium carrot, sliced (about 1 cup)

1 teaspoon rice wine

$^1/_4$ cup (60 ml) chicken or vegetable stock (made from chicken or vegetable bouillon cubes)

1 teaspoon light soy sauce

1 tablespoon oyster sauce

$^1/_2$ teaspoon sugar

$^1/_4$ teaspoon pepper

$^1/_2$ teaspoon cornstarch stirred into 1 teaspoon water

1 teaspoon sesame oil

1 Heat 3 tablespoons of the olive oil in a wok and fry the tofu until both sides are golden brown, 2–3 minutes on each side. Remove from the wok and drain.

2 In the same wok, heat the remaining 1 tablespoon of olive oil. Sprinkle in the salt and stir-fry the garlic until aromatic, about 1 minute. Stir in the grated ginger, mushrooms and carrot and stir-fry for 30 seconds.

3 Carefully add the tofu, then sizzle in the wine. Pour in the chicken or vegetable stock, soy sauce, oyster sauce, sugar, pepper and cornstarch. Mix carefully, then simmer covered over low heat for 15 minutes. Pour in the sesame oil, mix well, then serve hot.

Serves 2
Preparation time: 20 mins
Cooking time: 30 mins

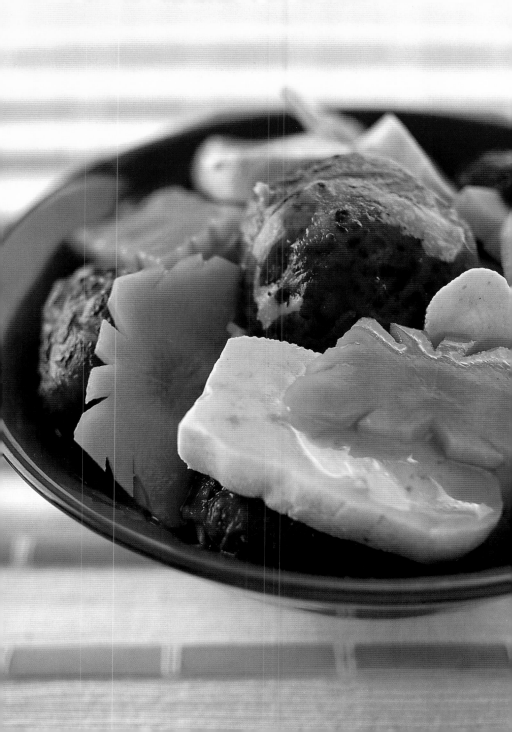

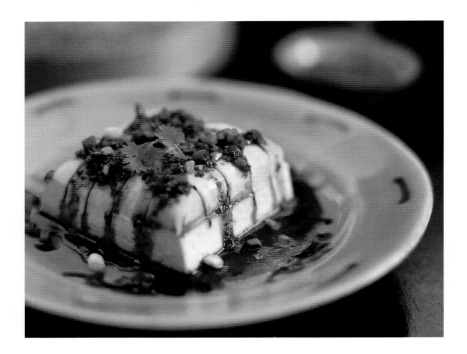

Poached Tofu with Spicy Sauce (China)

8 cups (2 liters) water
10 oz (300 g) medium or firm tofu
1 tablespoon chopped garlic
1 tablespoon finely chopped ginger
3 scallions, chopped
2 teaspoons chopped fresh cilantro (coriander leaves)

Sauce
1 tablespoon sesame oil
1 tablespoon chili oil
1 tablespoon soy sauce
1 teaspoon black pepper
$^1/_2$ teaspoon salt
1 teaspoon sugar

1 Bring the water to the boil in a medium pot, carefully add the tofu cake, reduce the heat and simmer for 4 minutes. Remove with a slotted spoon and drain. Alternatively, place the tofu in a steamer and steam for 4 minutes.
2 Mix all the Sauce ingredients well and set aside.
3 Place the garlic, ginger, and scallions in a bowl, then pour in the Sauce and mix thoroughly. Place the tofu in the center of a small serving dish. Make 4 cuts across the top of the tofu in both directions, cutting no more than halfway deep. Drizzle the sauce mixture evenly over the tofu and serve.

Serves 4
Preparation time: 10 mins
Cooking time: 5 mins

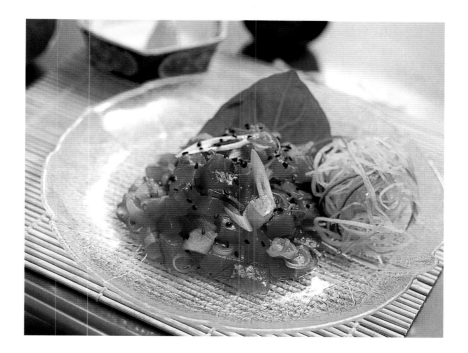

Tuna and Onion Appetizer (Japan)

2 tablespoons sliced baby leek
1 baby cucumber (about 4 oz/110 g) julienned
2 fresh *shiso* or large basil leaves, shredded
1$^1/_2$ teaspoons grated ginger
14 oz (400 g) fresh sashimi-quality tuna
Black sesame seeds (optional)

Ginger Dipping Sauce
1$^1/_2$ teaspoons grated ginger
Soy sauce

1 Place the sliced leeks in a small bowl of cold water and soak for 5 minutes. Drain and pat dry with paper towels.

2 Place the sliced leeks and shredded *shiso* leaves in a small bowl and chop. Add half of the ginger and toss to combine. Dice the tuna and toss carefully with the leek mixture.

3 To prepare the Ginger Dipping Sauce, divide the ginger between 4 small sauce bowls and top with soy sauce to taste.

4 Divide the tuna and cucumber between 4 dishes and arrange side-by-side. Sprinkle with black sesame seeds, if desired. Serve with Ginger Dipping Sauce.

Serves 4
Preparation time: **12–15 mins**

Diced Tofu with Vegetables (China)

8 oz (225 g) firm tofu, finely diced
$1/_4$ teaspoon fine salt
$1/_2$ cup (125 ml) oil
1 teaspoon finely chopped shallots
1 teaspoon finely chopped garlic
4 tablespoons dried shrimp, soaked and finely chopped
2 Chinese sausages (about 2 oz/60 g), diced
2 water chestnuts, peeled and diced
4 fresh Chinese or shiitake mushrooms, cubed
$1/_2$ small carrot, diced (about $1/_4$ cup/30 g)
2 tablespoons chopped preserved Chinese vegetable (page 6)
$1/_4$ cup (40 g) diced green or red bell peppers (capsicum)
1 chili, seeds removed and finely chopped
1 teaspoon rice wine
$1/_4$ cup (60 ml) chicken or vegetable stock (from chicken or vegetable bouillon cubes)
1 tablespoon oyster sauce
1–2 teaspoons soy sauce
1 teaspoon sugar
$1/_4$ teaspoon freshly ground black pepper
1 teaspoon sesame oil
2–3 large lettuce leaves, for serving
2 tablespoons chopped fresh cilantro (coriander leaves), to garnish

1 Sprinkle the diced tofu with the salt.

2 Heat the oil in a wok and deep-fry the tofu until golden, 2–3 minutes. Remove the tofu and drain.

3 Discard all but 1 tablespoon of the oil in the wok and stir-fry the shallots and garlic until fragrant, about 1 minute. Stir in the dried shrimp, Chinese sausages, water chestnuts, mushrooms and carrot, then stir-fry for 2 minutes.

4 Add the tofu, preserved Chinese vegetable, bell peppers and chili. Pour in the wine, then add the chicken or vegetable stock and the remaining ingredients. Stir briskly until evenly mixed. Divide among the lettuce leaves and serve garnished with the chopped cilantro.

Chinese sausages or lap cheong, *are widely available in unrefrigerated packages of various sizes in Asian food shops and well-stocked supermarkets. Made chiefly of pork, they are similar to salami and have a salty and slightly sweet taste. A similar quantity of diced bacon can be substituted if necessary.*

Serves 2–3
Preparation time: 30 mins
Cooking time: 20 mins

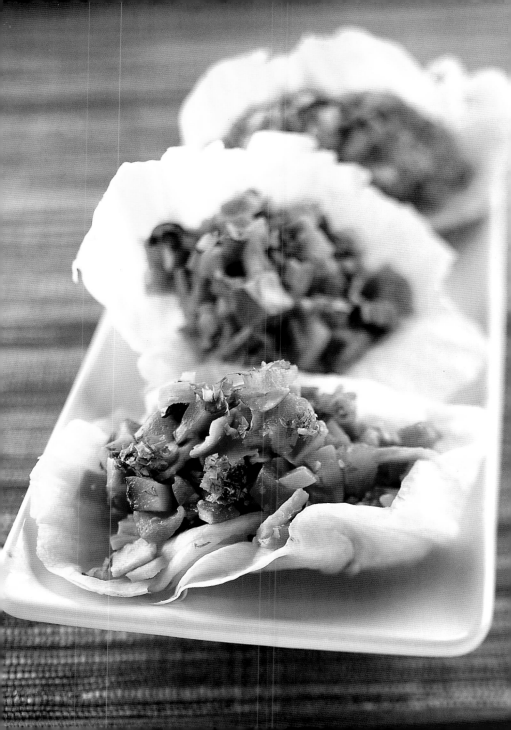

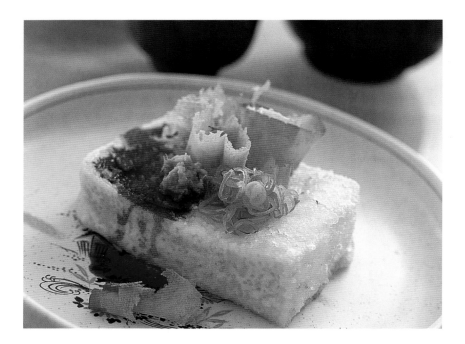

Deep-fried Tofu Appetizer (Japan)

10 oz (300 g) firm tofu
1 teaspoon cornstarch,
  for coating
Oil for deep-frying
1 tablespoon finely grated
  fresh ginger
1 tablespoon thinly sliced
  scallions
3 tablespoons bonito
  flakes or shaved bonito
Dark soy sauce, for
  serving

Serves 4
Preparation time: **10 mins**
Cooking time: **5 mins**

1 Drain the tofu and cut into 4 pieces widthwise.
Place each piece between 2 clean tea towels and gently
place a light weight on top, to help press out the
excess liquid. Let stand for 5 minutes.
2 Remove the weight from the tofu and dust the slices
with cornstarch, shaking lightly to remove the excess.
3 Heat the oil in a frying pan or wok over high heat.
Deep-fry the tofu slices until lightly browned, about
3–4 minutes each side, then drain on paper towels.
4 Serve immediately in small dishes topped with the
ginger, scallions and bonito flakes. Serve with soy
sauce on the side.

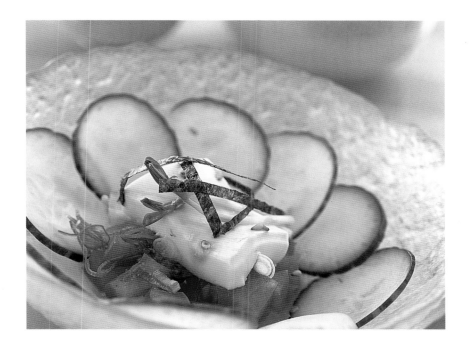

Fresh Tofu Appetizer (Japan)

10 oz (300 g) silken tofu
1 medium tomato (about 8 oz/250 g), finely diced
2 baby cucumbers (about 8 oz/220 g), thinly sliced
2 tablespoons finely sliced scallion
1 teaspoon white miso
2 teaspoons sesame oil
2 teaspoons rice wine vinegar
1 teaspoon sugar
1 teaspoon water
$^1/_2$ cup radish sprouts
1 sheet *nori*, toasted (see page 6), cut in half, then into thin strips
1 teaspoon sesame seeds, toasted

1 Drain the tofu and slice it in half lengthwise. Cut it into thick pieces and lay on a serving plate.
2 Gently combine the tomato, cucumber and scallions in a small bowl. Arrange the vegetables on individual serving plates or a single serving dish. Arrange the tofu on top.
3 In a small bowl, combine the miso, sesame oil, vinegar, sugar and water. Spoon over the tofu and vegetables. Top with radish sprouts and *nori*, sprinkle with sesame seeds and serve.

Serves 4
Preparation time: **10 mins**

Japanese Stir-fried
Mixed Vegetables (Japan)

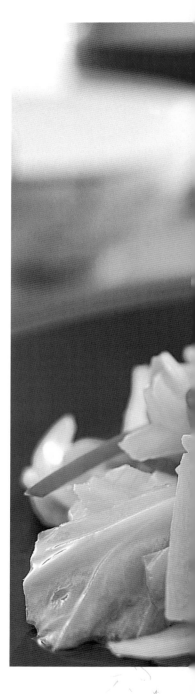

1 tablespoon Japanese sesame oil (see page 6)
1 small brown or yellow onion, cut into thin wedges
  (about $^3/_4$ cup)
1 small carrot, sliced into strips (about $^3/_4$ cup)
1 large green bell pepper (capsicum), sliced into strips
  (about 1 cup)
1 tablespoon finely chopped garlic
1 heaped teaspoon freshly grated ginger
10 snow peas ($^1/_2$ cup/50 g), tops and tails removed
1 head cabbage, shredded (about 4 cups)
1 cup (80 g) beansprouts, soaked in water and drained
2 tablespoons sake
$^1/_4$ teaspoon *dashi* powder or $^1/_4$ teaspoon chicken
  stock powder dissolved in 1 tablespoon water
4 teaspoons soy sauce

1 Heat the oil in a large frying pan or wok over high
heat and stir-fry the onion and carrot until onion is
transparent, about 2 minutes. Add the bell pepper
and continue stir-frying for another 2 minutes.
2 Add the garlic, ginger and snow peas and stir-fry
until fragrant, about 1 minute.
3 Add the cabbage and beansprouts and fry until the
cabbage starts to wilt, about 2 minutes.
4 Add the sake, *dashi* mixture and soy sauce, and stir-
fry until the cooking liquid is evaporated and the
vegetables are tender. Serve immediately.

Serves 4
Preparation time: **20 mins**
Cooking time: **10 mins**

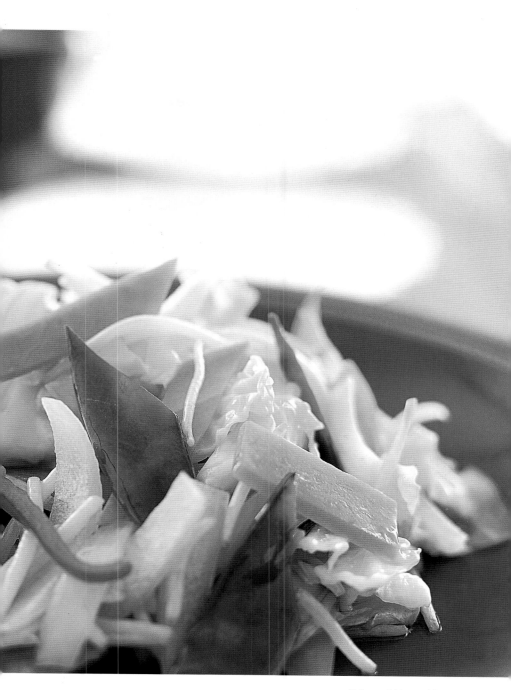

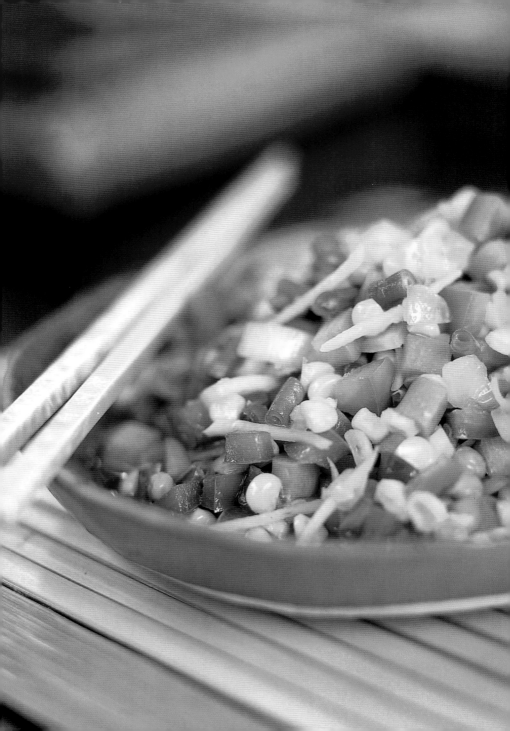

Mixed Diced Vegetables (China)

1 cup fresh or frozen
green peas
2 tablespoons oil
8 oz (225 g) fresh or
frozen corn kernels
(about $1^1/_2$ cups)
2 medium carrots, diced
(about $1^1/_2$ cups)
1 large green bell pepper
(capsicum), diced
(about $1^1/_2$ cups)
1 large onion (white,
yellow or red), diced
(about $1^1/_2$ cups)
5 oz (150 g) fresh or
frozen green beans,
tops and tails removed,
cut into short lengths
(about $1^1/_4$ cups)
2 tablespoons finely
chopped fresh ginger
1 teaspoon Sichuan
pepper-salt powder
(see page 6)

Sauce
1 tablespoon soy sauce
1 tablespoon water
1 teaspoon sugar
$^1/_2$ teaspoon salt
1 teaspoon sesame oil

1 Remove the green peas from their pods if using fresh
peas, or defrost the peas if frozen.

2 Combine the Sauce ingredients and set aside.

3 Heat the oil in a wok and, when hot, stir-fry the
corn, carrots, bell peppers, onions, green beans and
ginger for 2 minutes.

4 Add the peas, and continue to cook for another
1–2 minutes.

5 Add the Sauce, reduce the heat and cook slowly for
3–4 minutes, then add the Sichuan pepper-salt powder and stir for 1 more minute to completely blend
the flavors. Serve immediately.

Serves 4
Preparation time: **15 mins**
Cooking time: **10 mins**

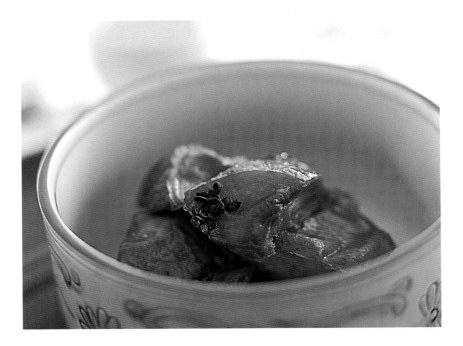

Glazed Sweet Potato Chunks (Japan)

2 medium sweet
potatoes (about
10 oz/300 g), washed
1 tablespoon oil
4 teaspoons *mirin*
1 teaspoon rice wine
vinegar
1 teaspoon soy sauce
2 teaspoons honey
1 teaspoon black sesame
seeds, to garnish

Serves 4
Preparation time: **10 mins**
Cooking time: **25 mins**

1 Place the sweet potatoes in a medium pan and cover with water. Bring to the boil, then reduce the heat to medium and cook until tender when pierced with a fork, about 15 minutes. Drain and set aside to cool.
2 Peel the potatoes thickly with a knife, removing skin and about $1/_8$ in (2 mm) of flesh. Cut into bite-sized pieces.
3 Heat the oil in a frying pan over medium heat. Add the sweet potatoes and stir-fry until the surface just starts to color, 3–4 minutes. Add the *mirin*, vinegar, soy sauce and honey, and cook until the liquid is reduced and starts to form a light caramel glaze around the surface of the potato, about 1 minute. Remove from the heat, sprinkle with the sesame seeds and serve as a snack or side dish.

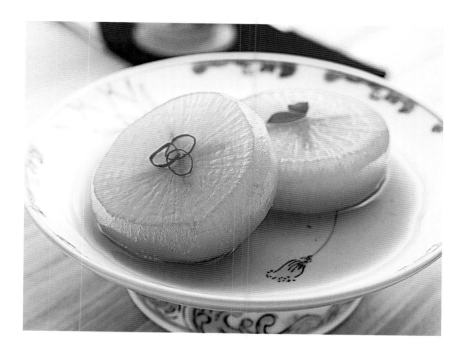

Braised Daikon (Japan)

1 daikon (about 1–1$^1/_4$
lbs/450–550 g)
1 teaspoon dashi
powder dissolved in 4
cups (1 liter) water
2 teaspoons sugar
2 tablespoons soy sauce
4 teaspoons sake
3 tablespoons *mirin*

Serves 4
Preparation time: **10 mins**
Cooking time: **3 hours**

1 Slice the daikon into 8 thick sections widthwise and remove the skin and thick outer layer. Cut a thin strip on an angle from the top and bottom edge of each piece. Cut a shallow cross into the top on one side.
2 Place the daikon into a medium saucepan with the dashi mixture, sugar, soy sauce and sake. Bring to the boil, removing any impurities from the surface with a spoon or paper towel. Boil for 10 minutes, then reduce the heat and simmer covered until daikon is tender and lightly browned, about 2$^1/_2$ hours.
3 Remove the cover and gently stir in the *mirin*. Let stand for 10 minutes before serving in small bowls with a little of the cooking liquid.

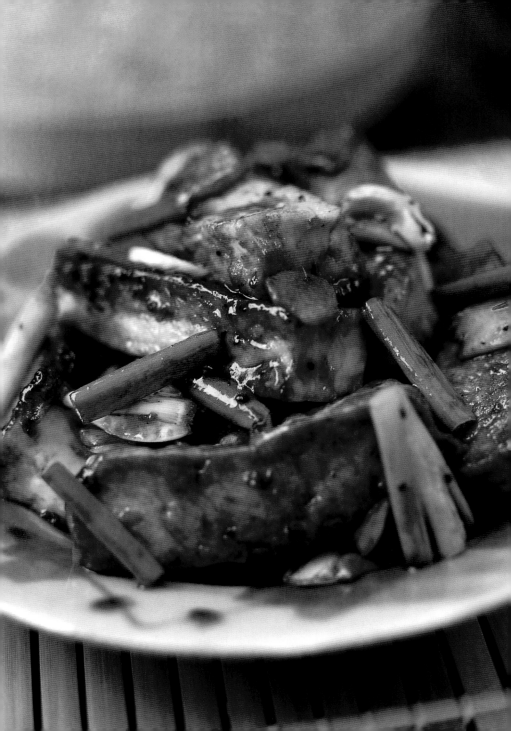

Homestyle Red-braised Tofu (China)

There are probably as many ways to prepare *hung shao* (red-braised) tofu, as there are cooks in China. This traditional method of cooking tofu, which by itself is a very bland food, allows the manifold flavors of the seasonings and sauce to penetrate the tofu, rendering this potent source of vegetable protein into a delicious dish. Each time you cook this dish, try a slightly different blend of flavors and proportions until you discover the style that best suits your taste.

5–6 dried Chinese mushrooms
1 lb (450 g) firm tofu
3 tablespoons oil
2 dried red chilies, cut in half, seeds and white membranes removed (optional)
4–5 large cloves garlic, skins removed and smashed
6 slices ginger
1 whole star anise (optional)
6 scallions, cut into 2-in (5-cm) lengths

Sauce
3 tablespoons soy sauce
2 tablespoons rice wine
1 tablespoon sesame oil
1 tablespoon sugar
$1/2$ teaspoon salt
$1/2$ teaspoon freshly ground black pepper
1 teaspoon cornstarch dissolved in $1/2$ cup (125 ml) water or chicken stock (made from chicken bouillon cubes)

1 Soak the mushrooms in warm water for about 20 minutes to soften, then drain. Remove and discard the stems, cut the mushrooms in half and set aside.
2 Cut the tofu into bite-sized cubes. Place in colander to drain.
3 Combine all the Sauce ingredients and set aside.
4 Heat the oil in a wok or large frying pan until hot, but not smoking. Add the chilies, if using, then the tofu, turning gently with a spatula until all the pieces are coated with oil and shaking the pan occasionally to prevent sticking. Fry until the tofu just begins to turn yellow but is not brown or crispy.
5 Add the mushrooms, garlic, ginger, star anise and half the scallions and stir-fry gently for 1–2 minutes.
6 Add the Sauce and stir carefully to blend. Cover the wok, lower the heat and braise for 5–6 minutes, adding a few tablespoons of water if the Sauce becomes too dry.
7 Add the remaining scallions to the wok and transfer to a serving dish.

Serves 4
Preparation time: 15 mins
Cooking time: 15 mins

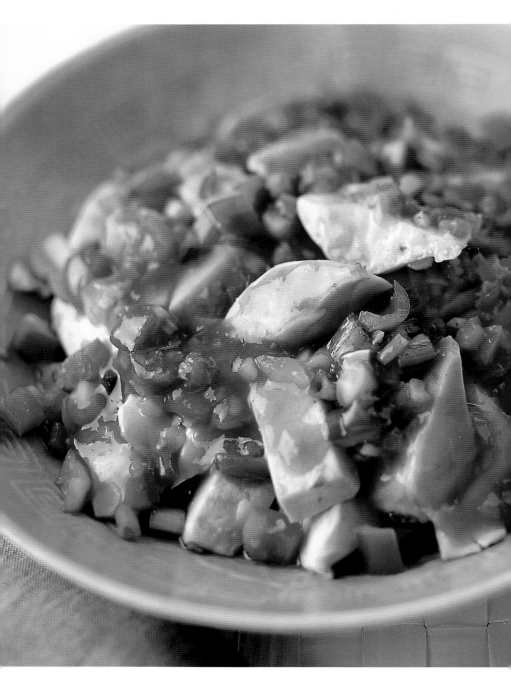

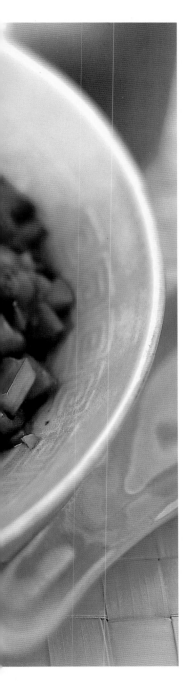

Vegetarian Ma Po Tofu (China)

10 oz (300 g) soft tofu, diced (about 1³/₄ cups)
2 tablespoons oil
2 teaspoons finely chopped garlic
1 red chili, seeds removed and thinly sliced
1 tablespoon hot broad bean paste
2 tablespoons preserved Chinese vegetable (see page
    6), chopped
1 teaspoon wine
¹/₄ cup (60 ml) chicken or vegetable stock (made
    from chicken or vegetable bouillon cubes)
1 tablespoon soy sauce
1 teaspoon sugar
¹/₄ teaspoon freshly ground black pepper
¹/₂ cup (80 g) diced green bell pepper (capsicum)
2 teaspoons cornstarch stirred in 2 teaspoons water
1 teaspoon sesame oil
1 scallion, thinly sliced, to garnish

1 Bring a small saucepan of water to the boil. Blanch the cubed tofu for about 4 minutes. Rinse and drain.
2 Heat the oil in a wok and stir-fry the garlic and chili for about 1 minute. Add the broad bean paste and stir-fry until aromatic, about 1 more minute, then stir in the preserved Chinese vegetable.
3 Pour in the wine, then add the chicken or vegetable stock, soy sauce, sugar and pepper, then mix to combine. Add the tofu and capsicum, stirring carefully, then simmer over low heat for 2 minutes.
4 Add the cornstarch mixture and stir gently until the sauce thickens. Sprinkle with the sesame oil and serve hot, garnished with the chopped scallions.

Hot broad bean paste (do ban jian or toban djan), or chili bean sauce, is a Sichuan-style chili sauce made from chilies and fermented broad beans. It is used to add heat to cooked dishes or as a dipping sauce.

Serves 2
Preparation time: **20 mins**
Cooking time: **20 mins**

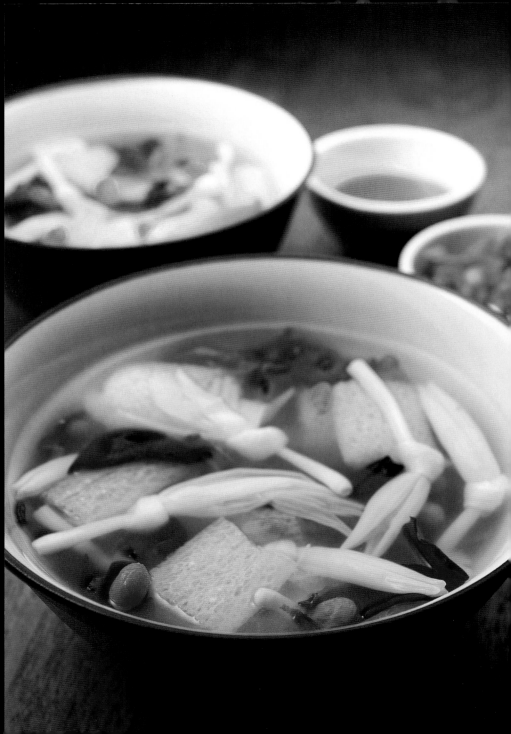

"Forget Your Troubles" Soup (China)

This is a soothing soup with cooling, calming medicinal properties. Its Chinese name translates as "forget your troubles" and is derived from the combined effects of the tiger lily buds, bamboo pith and wolfberry, which calm "liver fire" and relax the nervous system. Chinese vegetarian cuisine has a long tradition of blending beneficial medicinal herbs with ordinary food items to create dishes that nourish the body, correct imbalances and please the palate, all in one dish.

3¹/₄ cups (800 ml) vegetable or chicken stock (made from vegetable or chicken bouillon cubes)
¹/₂ teaspoon salt
1 tablespoon dried wolfberries
¹/₂ cup (50 g) dried tiger lily buds, bases trimmed, soaked in water 20 minutes and drained
6 pieces fresh or dried black wood ear mushrooms (if dried, soak in water for 20 minutes), cut into thick strips
8 pieces dried bamboo fungus, soaked in cool water for 20 minutes and snipped into ³/₄-in (4-cm) lengths (see note)
Seasonings and condiments for serving (see note)

1 Bring the vegetable or chicken stock to the boil with the salt, then add the wolfberries, and let water return to the boil. Add the tiger lily buds, wood ear mushrooms and bamboo fungus. Bring the soup to the boil. Cover, lower the heat and simmer for 3 minutes.
2 Serve hot.

Soups like this are traditionally served with a tray of seasonings and condiments so that each person can season the soup to their own personal taste. Try the following choices: sesame oil, red chili oil, Sichuan pepper-salt powder, chopped fresh cilantro (coriander leaves), chopped scallions, chopped basil leaves and chopped parsley.
Wolfberries, *the fruit of the Chinese boxthorn or matrimony vine, are available dried. They look and taste a bit like small red currants but are not as sweet.*
Dried bamboo fungus *is actually the dried pith of the bamboo plant. If necessary, substitute with finely julienned bamboo shoots.*
Dried tiger lily buds *are the unopened buds of a variety of Chinese day lily. The buds are soaked and their tough stems removed before use. All three ingredients are available at Asian food shops.*

Serves 4
Preparation time: 15 mins + 20 mins soaking time
Cooking time: 20 mins

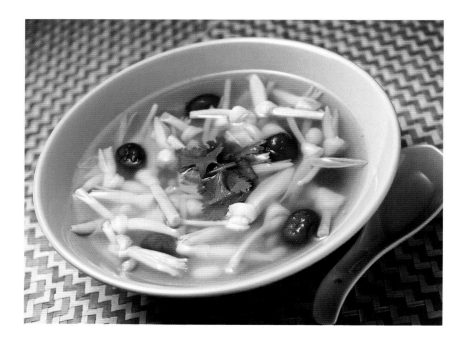

Tiger Lily and Soybean Soup (China)

6 cups (1¹/₂ liters) vegetable stock (made from vegetable bouillon cubes) or water
¹/₂ cup (100 g) dried soybeans, picked through for grit, rinsed and soaked overnight, then drained
¹/₂ cup (50 g) dried tiger lily buds (see page 43), washed, bases trimmed
6 Chinese red dates, washed, pits removed
2 slices ginger
1 teaspoon salt
1 tablespoon fresh cilantro (coriander leaves)

1 Bring the vegetable stock or water to the boil in a large pot, then add the soybeans. Return to the boil, then cover, lower heat and simmer gently for 1 hour.
2 Add the tiger lily buds and red dates. Bring the soup to the boil again and simmer for 15 minutes.
3 Add the salt and serve garnished with the cilantro.

At the end of the meal, there will be some soybeans remaining at the bottom of the bowl. Don't discard these. Instead, drain them from the soup, then heat 1 tablespoon oil in a wok to medium hot, throw in the cooked soybeans, 1 teaspoon sugar and 1 tablespoon soy sauce, and stir-fry for 1–2 minutes. This makes a delicious late-night snack!

Serves 4
Preparation time: **10 mins + overnight soaking**
Cooking time: **2 ¹/₄ hours**

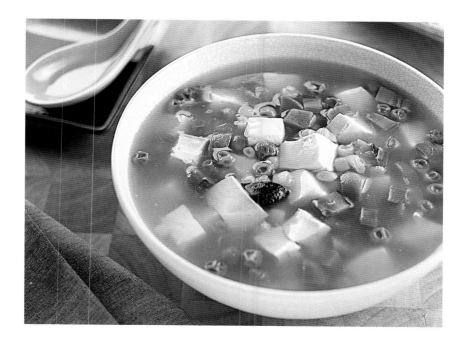

Sweet Corn and Tofu Chowder (China)

1 tablespoon oil
1 teaspoon rice wine
4 cups (1 liter) vegetable or chicken stock (made from bouillon cubes)
$1/2$ small carrot, diced
6 straw mushrooms, diced
6 fresh shiitake or Chinese mushrooms, diced
10 oz (300 g) soft tofu, diced
1 cup (200 g) fresh or frozen sweet corn
2 tablespoons green peas
1 teaspoon salt
2 tablespoons cornstarch dissolved in 2 table-spoons stock or water
$1/4$ teaspoon pepper
1 teaspoon sesame oil

1 Heat the oil in a wok or saucepan, then add the rice wine and let it sizzle before pouring in the chicken or vegetable stock. Bring to the boil.
2 Add the carrot and mushrooms and simmer for 5 minutes. Add the diced tofu and sweet corn, simmer another 5 minutes, then add the green peas and salt.
3 Add the cornstarch and stir until the soup thickens to the consistency of chowder. Add the pepper and sesame oil and serve hot.

Serves 2–4
Preparation time: 20 mins
Cooking time: 20 mins

Vegetable and Tofu Soup
(China)

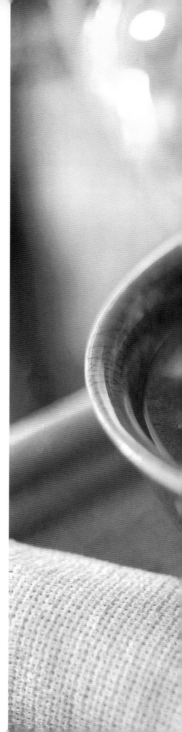

6 cups (1 1/2 liters) water
2 teaspoons salt
6–8 large or 12 small dried Chinese black mushrooms,
  soaked in hot water and drained
5 oz (140 g) fresh spinach, watercress, bok choy or
  similar greens
7 oz (200 g) soft tofu, cut into cubes
5 slices ginger, julienned
1/4 cup fresh cilantro (coriander leaves)

1 Bring the water to the boil in a large pot, then add the salt.
2 Cut away and discard the tough stems from the mushrooms, then cut the large mushrooms in half (leave small mushrooms whole, if using).
3 Wash and rinse the vegetables. Remove any tough or wilted stems, and separate the leaves.
4 Add the mushrooms to the boiling water, and let the water return to the boil, then add the tofu and ginger. Return to the boil over medium heat, cover, and simmer for about 20 minutes.
5 Add the vegetables and stir, return to the boil, then simmer for 2 more minutes.
6 Serve garnished with fresh cilantro.

Adding a few dashes of sesame oil to this soup gives it a rich, nutty aromatic flavor. Other popular table condiments for this soup are freshly ground black pepper, Sichuan pepper-salt powder and various chili sauces. You may also use other kinds of vegetables to make this soup. Broccoli is quite good (but be sure to peel the stems, which are bitter), or try cauliflower, cabbage, turnip and beansprouts.

Serves 4
Preparation time: 20 mins
Cooking time: 30 mins

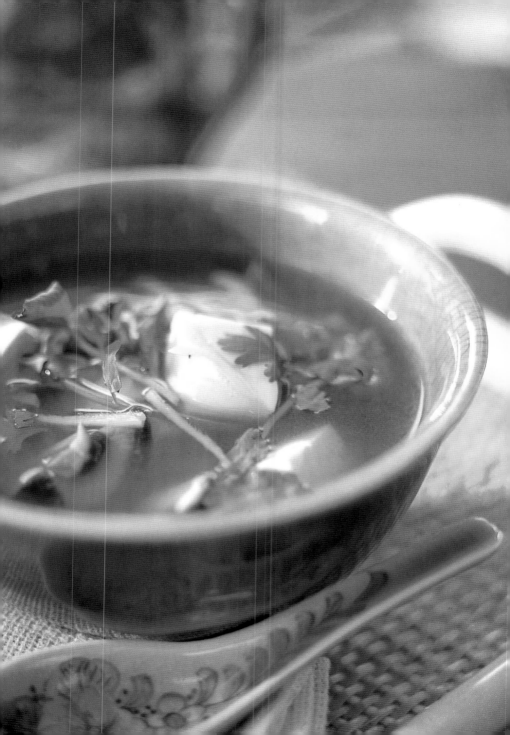

Spicy and Sour Soup with Shrimps and Pineapple (Vietnam)

This recipe produces a flavorful result and gives the shrimp added texture. The soup comes together quickly, so assemble all the ingredients before cooking.

1 lb (450 g) medium shrimp, peeled and deveined
1 teaspoon cornstarch for dusting
3 tablespoons oil
6 cups (1¹/₂ liters) chicken or fish stock (made from chicken or fish bouillon cubes)
1 tablespoon tamarind pulp soaked in ¹/₃ cup (80 ml) water (page 7)
2 large stalks celery, thinly sliced or julienned
1¹/₂ cups (350 g) peeled and cubed fresh ripe pineapple
1 large tomato, cut into wedges
8 pieces okra (ladies' fingers), sliced
2 red or green chilies, thinly sliced
2¹/₂ cups (200 g) beansprouts, rinsed
2 tablespoons fish sauce
1¹/₂ tablespoons sugar
¹/₂ teaspoon salt
2 shallots, peeled and minced
¹/₂ cup fresh cilantro (coriander leaves), to garnish
¹/₂ cup Thai basil, to garnish

1 Dust the shrimp with the cornstarch. Heat 2 tablespoons of the oil in a frying pan over medium heat and stir-fry the shrimp until pink, about 3 minutes. Remove from the heat and set aside.

2 In a large saucepan, heat the chicken or fish stock and tamarind juice over medium heat. Add the celery, pineapple, tomato, okra and chilies, then bring to the boil. Reduce the heat to low, add the beansprouts, and stir in the fish sauce, sugar and salt.

3 Heat the remaining oil in a frying pan and stir-fry the shallots until golden, about 4 minutes. Add the shrimp to the soup, stirring to combine well. Remove from the heat and serve, garnished with shallots and fresh cilantro and Thai basil leaves.

Serves 6–8
Preparation time: 15 mins
Cooking time: 10 mins

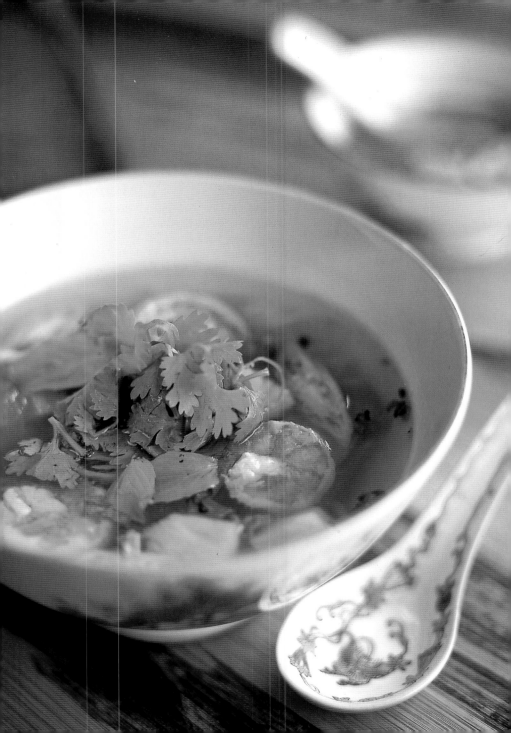

Fish Soup with Fennel (China)

According to Chinese medicine, this recipe provides a variety of therapeutic benefits, including eliminating phlegm from the body, strengthening spleen and stomach functions, and counteracting symptoms of colds and flu. Any type of white-fleshed saltwater fish may be used in this soup.

1 lb (450 g) fresh white-fleshed saltwater fish, such as sea bass, white marlin or swordfish
2 tablespoons white sesame seeds, dry roasted, then finely ground in a blender or food processor
2 tablespoons oil
6 cups (1 $^1/_2$ liters) boiling water or fish stock (made from fish bouillon cubes)
1 baby fennel bulb, halved, cored and finely sliced, leaves reserved to garnish (optional)

Seasoning
1 teaspoon soy sauce
1 teaspoon sugar
2 teaspoons ground fennel seeds
1 teaspoon salt

Serves 4
Preparation time: **20 mins**
Marinating time: **2 hours**
Cooking time: **10 mins**

1 Rinse the fish and pat dry with paper towels, then cut it into bite-sized pieces.
2 Place the sesame powder in a shallow bowl, then toss the fish pieces in the sesame powder until evenly coated. Cover the bowl and allow the fish to rest in the sesame powder for 2 hours.
3 Combine the Seasoning ingredients and set aside.
4 Heat the oil in a wok or large pot until hot and stir-fry the fish for 2 minutes, then immediately add the boiling water or fish stock. Return to the boil, then add the Seasoning and stir to mix.
5 Cover, reduce the heat and simmer for 5 minutes. Serve garnished with fennel slices and leaves, if desired.

You may also prepare this soup with **fresh shrimps** *that have been shelled and deveined. This is a good way to prepare fish or shrimps for people with digestive problems; the fennel and sesame aid digestion, and the water provides plenty of fluid to carry it through the digestive tract.*
Fennel bulbs *are stumpy plants with thick stems They have round bases that resemble large onions and have an aniseed taste. They are sold fresh in supermarkets. If fennel bulbs are not available, substitute with parsley.*

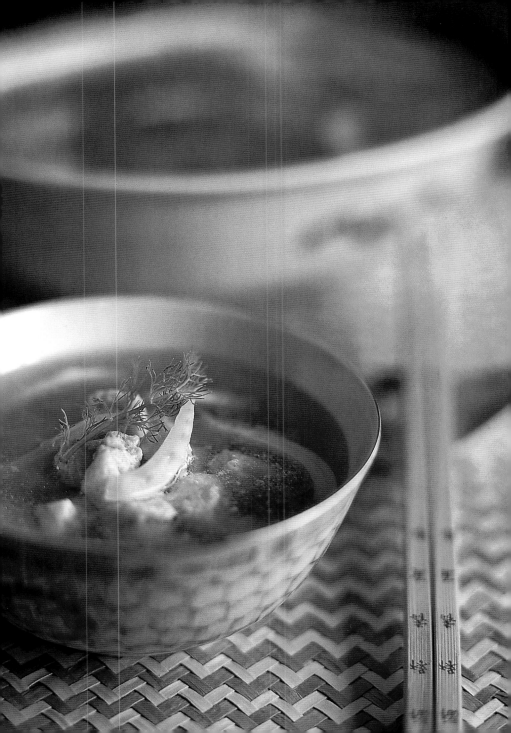

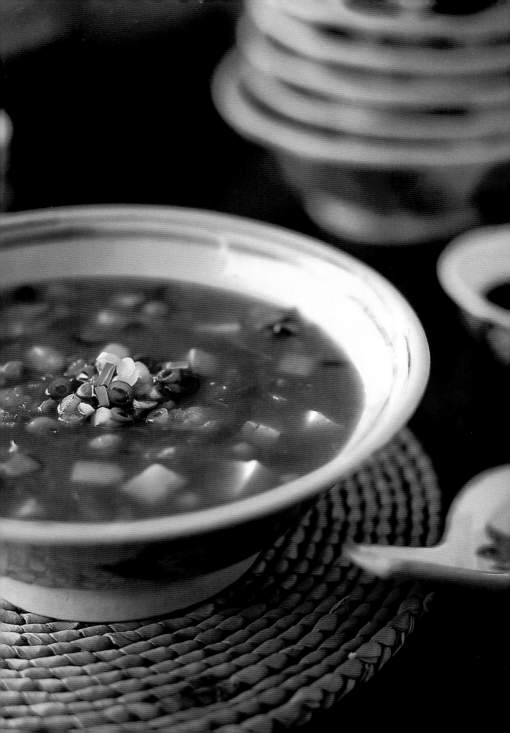

Sichuan Hot and Sour Soup (China)

$2^1/_2$ oz (75 g) boneless chicken breast
1 slice dark cured ham or prosciutto (about 30 g/ 1 oz)
1 cake dried or firm tofu
1 oz (30 g) canned or fresh bamboo shoots
1 small carrot
4 large fresh or dried shiitake mushrooms
1 oz (30 g) fresh or dried wood ear mushrooms
4 cups (1 liter) chicken stock or water (made from chicken bouillon cubes)
2 teaspoons salt
1 teaspoon sugar
$1/_2$ cup fresh or frozen green peas
2 eggs, well beaten
$1^1/_2$ tablespoons soy sauce
2 tablespoons vinegar
2 teaspoons sesame oil
$1/_2$ teaspoon freshly ground black pepper
$1/_2$ teaspoon ground Sichuan pepper
2 tablespoons cornstarch dissolved in 4 tablespoons cool water
$1/_4$ cup chopped fresh cilantro (coriander leaves)
6 slices ginger, julienned
4 scallions, chopped

1 Poach the chicken and ham in boiling water for 2 minutes, then drain and set aside to cool. Shred finely with fingers or a sharp knife and set aside.
2 Cut the dried or firm tofu, bamboo shoots, and carrot into small dice, and set aside.
3 If using dried mushrooms, soak them separately in hot water for 20 minutes and drain. Dice all the mushrooms, discarding the stems, and set aside.
4 Bring chicken or vegetable stock to the boil in a large pot. Add the salt, sugar, peas and the reserved meat and vegetables and stir well. Return to the boil, reduce the heat and simmer for 3 minutes.
5 Slowly drizzle the beaten eggs across the surface of the simmering soup and leave without stirring for 1 minute.
6 Add the soy sauce, vinegar, sesame oil, black pepper and Sichuan pepper, and stir to blend for 1 minute.
7 Stir the cornstarch and water again, then pour slowly into the simmering soup while stirring gently, and keep stirring until the soup thickens. Simmer 1 more minute, then turn off heat.
8 Serve garnished with cilantro, ginger and scallions.

In place of dried tofu, you can drain a cake of firm or medium tofu for 3–4 hours with a weight on top to help press out excess water. Cut the drained tofu into strips or cubes and add to the soup.
Adventurous cooks may wish to improvise using a variety of meats, seafoods and vegetables. For a vegetarian version, use vegetable stock or plain water rather than chicken stock. Eliminate the chicken and ham, and double the quantities of tofu and shiitake mushrooms. Possible condiments to go with this dish are red chili oil, sesame oil, Sichuan pepper-salt powder, minced fresh red chili and vinegar.

Serves 4
Preparation time: **30 mins**
Cooking time: **30 mins**

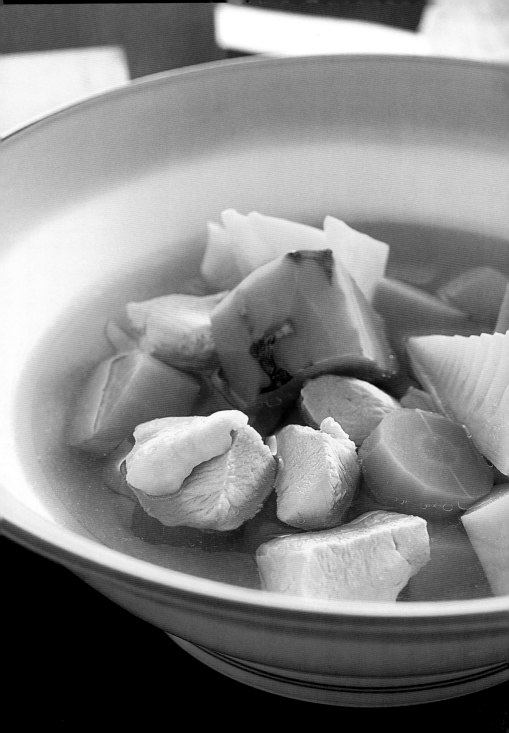

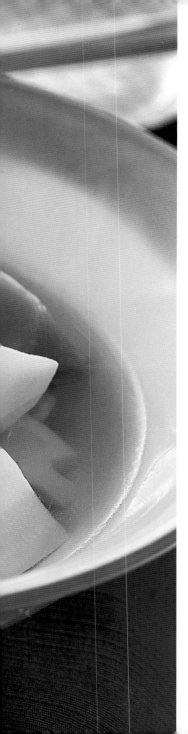

Savory Chicken and Vegetable Soup (Japan)

6 cups (1 1/2 liters) water
10 oz (300 g) boneless chicken meat, skin removed,
  cut into bite-sized pieces
1 large or 2 small carrots, cut into bite-sized chunks
8 oz (250 g) winter squash (such as butternut), skin
  and seeds removed, cut into chunks (about 2 cups)
6 oz (180 g) bamboo shoots, sliced into bite-sized
  chunks (about 1 1/2 cups)
3 teaspoons *dashi* powder
3 tablespoons soy sauce
3 tablespoons sake
3 tablespoons *mirin*

1 Bring the water to the boil in a large pot. Add the
chicken and cook over medium heat for 2 minutes,
removing any impurities from the surface with a
spoon or paper towel.
2 Add the carrot, pumpkin and bamboo shoots.
3 Stir in the *dashi* powder, soy sauce, sake and *mirin*.
Return to the boil and cover the pan. Boil rapidly for
5 minutes, then reduce heat and simmer covered until
vegetables are tender, about 20 minutes.
4 Let stand for 10 minutes before serving the vegetables in small bowls with a little of the cooking liquid.

Serves 4
Preparation time: **20 mins**
Cooking time: **40 mins**

Tofu Soup with Beansprouts (Thailand)

4 cups (1 liter) chicken or vegetable stock (made from chicken or vegetable bouillon cubes)
1 lb (450 g) soft tofu, cubed
1 cup (110 g) beansprouts
1 tablespoon preserved Chinese vegetable (see page 6), chopped
1 tablespoon fish sauce
$^1/_2$ teaspoon salt
$^1/_2$ teaspoon freshly ground white pepper
1 scallion, thinly sliced
1 tablespoon coarsely chopped fresh cilantro (coriander leaves)

1 Bring the chicken or vegetable stock to the boil over medium heat, then add the tofu, stirring to prevent it from sticking.
2 Add the sprouts when the soup returns to the boil. Cook for 2–3 minutes, then add the remaining ingredients, stirring well to combine. Serve immediately.

Serves 4
Preparation time: **10 mins**
Cooking time: **10 mins**

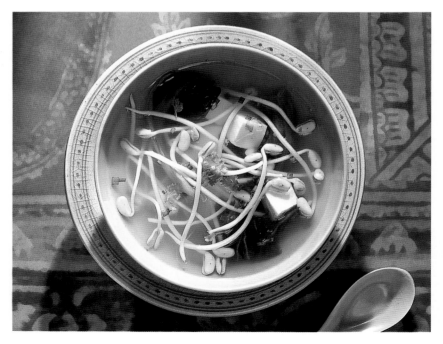

Chicken and Ginseng Soup (China)

$^1/_2$ chicken, about 1 lb
(450 g), skin and fat
discarded
10 oz (300 g) lean pork
2 tablespoons sliced
American ginseng
3 dried Chinese red dates,
washed and pitted
1 slice ginger, lightly
smashed
8 cups (2 liters) water
1 teaspoon salt

Serves 2–4
Preparation time: 30 mins
Cooking time: 2 hours

1 Bring a pot of water to the boil. Blanch the chicken in the boiling water for 1–2 minutes, then rinse and drain. Blanch the pork the same way.
2 Place all the ingredients, except the salt, in a large pot and bring to the boil, then lower the heat and simmer for two hours. Add the salt and serve hot.

American ginseng is one of the less expensive varieties of this root with a divided shape that resembles a human body. It is considered to be a general, all-healing tonic, and is available dried in Asian food shops or where Chinese medicines are sold. Fresh roots are sometimes available in Asian food shops that sell fresh vegetables.

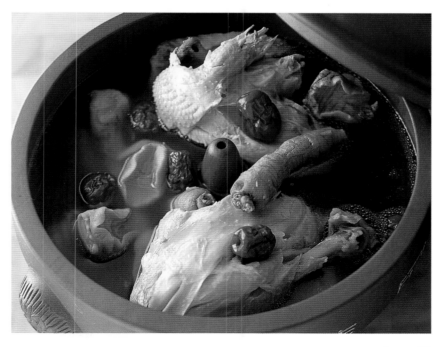

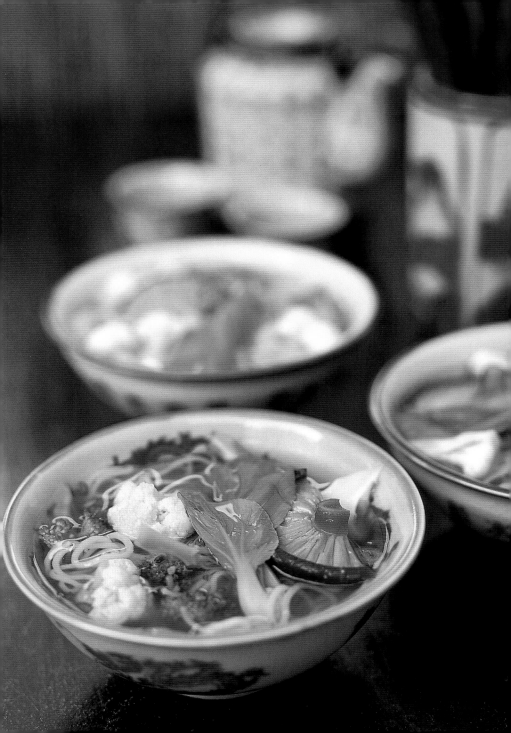

Noodles in Vegetable Broth (China)

12–16 cups (3–4 liters) water, to cook noodles

6 cups (1 1/2 liters) water, with 1 teaspoon salt, to make vegetable broth

12 dried shiitake or Chinese mushrooms, soaked in 1 cup (250 ml) hot water

8 oz (250 g) dried or 1 lb (450 g) fresh wheat noodles

8 florets fresh broccoli, stems peeled, each cut into pieces (2 cups)

8 florets fresh cauliflower, stems peeled, each cut into pieces (2 cups)

1 large or 2 small heads bok choy, washed with leaves separated

Seasonings

3 scallions, finely chopped

4 teaspoons sesame oil

2 teaspoons sugar

2 teaspoons Sichuan pepper-salt powder

Serves 4
Preparation time: 30 mins
Cooking time: 30 mins

1 Bring the water for the noodles and the vegetable broth to the boil in separate pots.

2 Drain mushrooms, adding the soaking water to the pot for the vegetable broth. Discard the mushroom stems and cut each mushroom in half.

3 Boil the noodles and cook until done, about 5–7 minutes for dried noodles (check the label for instructions), or about 30 seconds for fresh noodles. Drain the noodles and divide them among four serving bowls.

4 Add the mushrooms to the boiling salted water and simmer for 10 minutes. Add the broccoli and cauliflower and simmer for 2 more minutes, then add the bok choy leaves and simmer 1 more minute. Turn off the heat.

5 Divide the Seasonings among the bowls of noodles and mix to combine.

6 With a slotted spoon or chopsticks, distribute the cooked vegetables evenly among the four bowls of noodles, then ladle enough broth from the pot to fill each bowl. Serve hot.

This dish is usually prepared with ordinary Chinese wheat noodles, dried or fresh, but any sort of noodles, such as rice noodles or bean thread vermicelli can be used as long as you follow the cooking instructions on the package labels. And, of course, you may substitute any combination of vegetables that suits your tastes and nutritional requirements.

Soba Noodles in Sweet Soy Broth (Japan)

3 tablespoons dried *wakame* seaweed
1 lb (450 g) dried soba noodles
1 leek, white part only, very thinly sliced
4–6 tablespoons red pickled ginger
4–6 eggs (optional)
$^1/_4$ cup (60 g) sugar
1$^1/_3$ cups (330 ml) *mirin*
5 teaspoons *dashi* powder dissolved in 4 cups (1 liter) water
1 cup soy sauce
$^1/_4$ teaspoon Japanese seven-spice chili powder (optional)

1 Soak the seaweed in cold water until reconstituted, about 5 minutes. Drain and set aside.

2 Cook the noodles according to the package instructions. Drain and rinse well in cold water to remove excess surface starch.

3 Divide the noodles between 4–6 medium bowls. Arrange the seaweed, leek and pickled ginger on top of the noodles, then crack an egg carefully into the center of each bowl.

4 Combine the sugar and *mirin* in a medium saucepan over medium heat and stir until the sugar is dissolved. Add the *dashi* mixture and soy sauce, then stir and bring to the boil.

5 Immediately pour the hot broth over the noodles and serve sprinkled with the seven-spice chili powder, if desired.

Serves 4–6
Preparation time: **10 mins**
Cooking time: **10 mins**

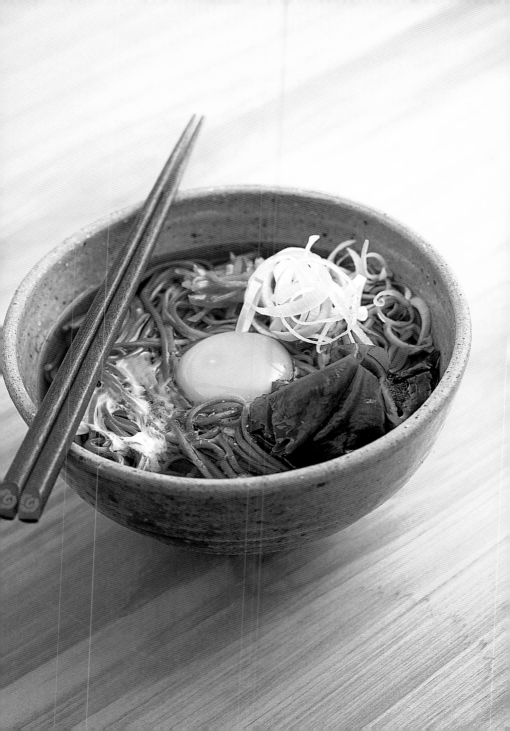

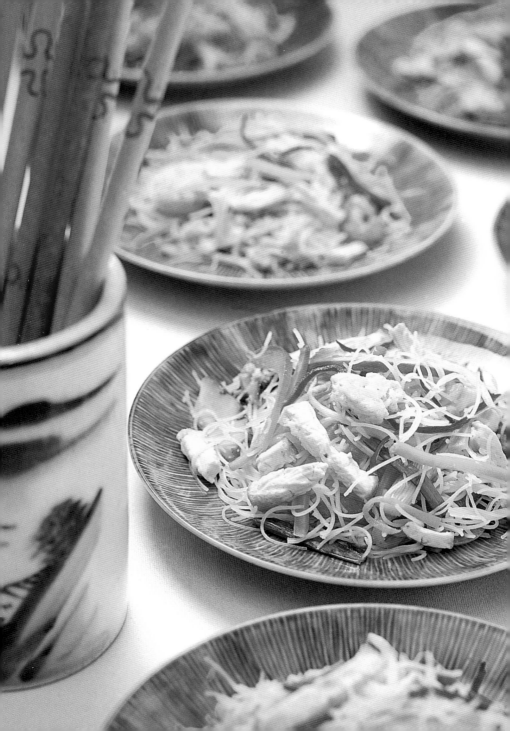

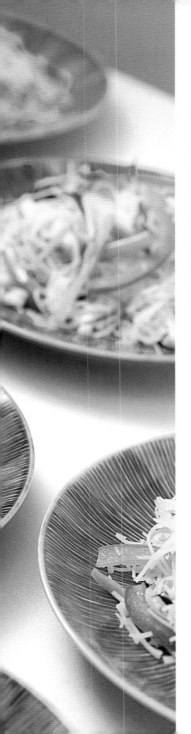

Vegetarian Rice Vermicelli
(Singapore)

4 tablespoons oil
1 medium onion, halved and thinly sliced
5 dried black Chinese mushrooms, soaked in hot water
  to soften, stems discarded, caps thinly sliced
2 teaspoons finely chopped garlic
1–2 large red chilies, thinly sliced
1 medium carrot, coarsely grated or sliced
1 medium green bell pepper (capsicum), julienned
7 oz (200 g) extra firm tofu, deep-fried until golden
  brown, then cut into strips
2 cups (160 g) beansprouts, washed and drained
2 eggs, lightly beaten
1 tablespoon soy sauce
10 oz (300 g) dried rice vermicelli, soaked in hot water
  to soften, then drained and cut in 4-in (10-cm) lengths
1 scallion, cut in $^3/_4$-in (2-cm) lengths
Bottled chili sauce or 1–2 small red chilies, sliced
2–3 small green limes, quartered, for serving

1 Heat the oil in a wok, then add the onion and stir-fry until it starts to soften, about 2 minutes. Add the mushrooms, garlic and chilies and stir-fry for 1 minute. Add the carrot and bell pepper then stir-fry over high heat for 2 minutes.
2 Add the tofu and beansprouts and stir-fry for 30 seconds. Pour in the egg and leave until it starts to set, about 15 seconds, then stir vigorously. Add the soy sauce and stir to combine.
3 Add the rice vermicelli and sliced scallions and stir-fry until well mixed and heated through, about 1 minute. Transfer to a serving dish and serve with chili sauce or sliced chilies and lime.

Serves 4–6
Preparation time: **20 mins**
Cooking time: **10 mins**

Chicken Noodle Soup (Vietnam)

Traditionally, this meal-in-a-bowl soup is made with beef and beef bones, but the Vietnamese have perfected a lighter non-beef version using chicken. This soup is popular at any time of day or night and is often enjoyed for breakfast in Vietnam.

1 whole chicken, about (3 lbs/1$^1/_4$ kg)
8 cups (2 liters) chicken stock (made from chicken bouillon cubes)
1 cinnamon stick
3 scallions
1 tablespoon freshly grated ginger
1$^1/_2$ teaspoons salt
1 teaspoon sugar
1$^1/_2$ tablespoons fish sauce
10 oz (300 g) dried rice stick noodles (about 4$^1/_2$ cups cooked noodles)
3 cups (240 g) fresh beansprouts, blanched
2 tablespoons fresh cilantro (coriander leaves)
$^1/_2$ yellow onion, very thinly sliced crosswise (optional)
3 scallions sliced into 1-in (2$^1/_2$-cm) pieces for serving
1 cup fresh Thai basil leaves
1 lime, cut into wedges (optional)

1 Place the chicken and the chicken stock in a large stockpot with the cinnamon, scallions, fresh ginger, salt and sugar then bring to the boil over medium heat. Reduce the heat to low and continue cooking for 1 more hour. Add the fish sauce and set aside.

2 Meanwhile, to cook the noodles, bring a large pot of water to the boil, put in the noodles and cook until tender, about 8 minutes. Remove from the heat, drain, rinse in cold water and set aside.

3 Half an hour before serving, remove the chicken from the stock and when it is cool enough to handle, shred the meat by hand and set aside.

4 To serve, place a handful of noodles in a large soup bowl. Top with some beansprouts and shredded chicken. Garnish with the fresh cilantro leaves, onion slices, if desired, scallions and basil. Ladle in the soup and sprinkle with fresh lime juice, if desired. Add more fish sauce to taste, if desired. Repeat the process for each serving.

Serves 8
Preparation time: 20 mins
Cooking time: 1 hour 20 mins

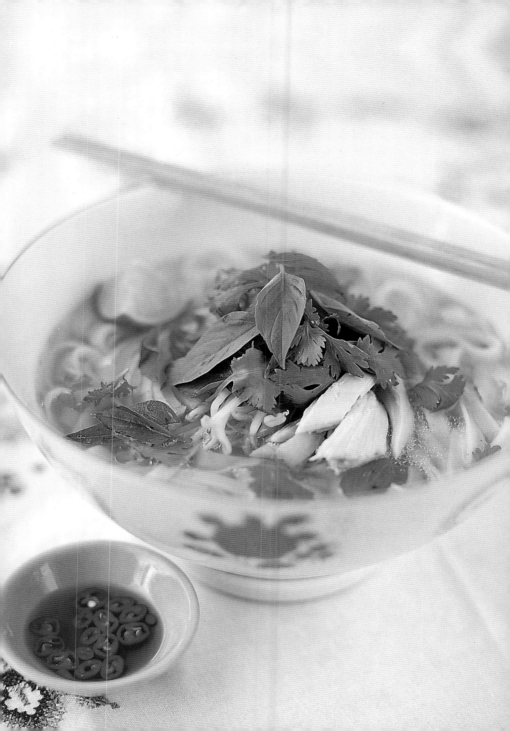

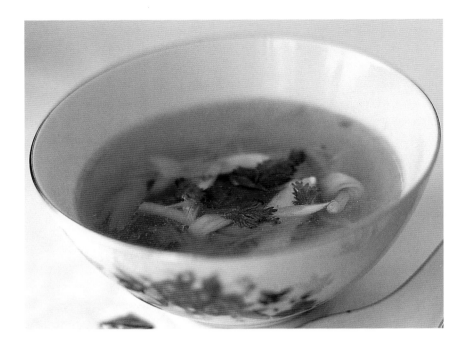

Bean Thread Noodle Soup (Vietnam)

1 1/2 oz (40 g) dried
    bean thread vermicelli
20 tiger lily buds
5 cups (1 1/4 liters) chick-
    en stock (made from
    chicken bouillon cubes)
    or water
1 boneless chicken
    breast, cut into strips,
    (about 1 cup)
2 tablespoons fish sauce
1/2 teaspoon salt
1/2 teaspoon freshly
    ground black pepper
1 scallion, thinly sliced
1 tablespoon coarsely
    chopped fresh cilantro
    (coriander leaves)

1 Soak the dried bean thread noodles and tiger lily buds, separately, in warm water for 30 minutes. Drain the noodles, divide them into three portions and set aside. Drain the tiger lily buds, remove the hard tips, tie a knot in each bud and set aside.

2 Heat the chicken stock or water in a large pot over medium heat. Stir in the tiger lily buds, then add the chicken meat, fish sauce, salt and black pepper. Bring the soup to the boil, then lower the heat and simmer until the chicken is cooked, about 10 minutes.

3 Add the bean thread noodles to the soup. When heated through, about 1 minute, remove from the heat and serve immediately, garnished with the sliced scallions and fresh cilantro leaves.

Serves 4
Preparation time: **10 mins + 30 mins soaking**
Cooking time: **25 mins**

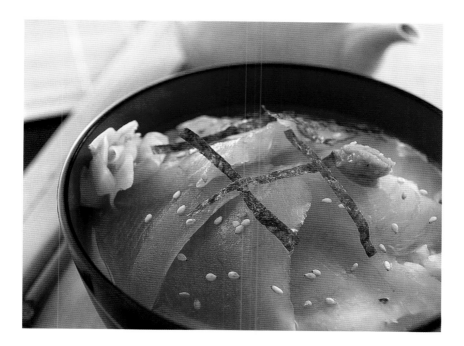

Sashimi Tuna Rice Bowl (Japan)

5 cups freshly cooked Japanese rice
$^1/_2$ teaspoon *dashi* powder dissolved in 1$^1/_2$ cups (375 ml) water
3 tablespoons soy sauce
3 tablespoons *mirin*
2 teaspoons *wasabi*
1 sheet *nori*, toasted and cut in thin strips
12 oz (350 g) fresh, sashimi-quality tuna, thinly sliced
2 tablespoons red pickled ginger
$^1/_2$ teaspoon sesame seeds

1 Divide the rice among 4 medium bowls.
2 Combine the *dashi* mixture, soy sauce, *mirin* and *wasabi* in a small bowl, then divide into four equal portions and pour over each bowl of rice. Sprinkle with the *nori*, reserving a little for garnish.
3 Arrange the tuna on top of the rice and serve garnished with the reserved *nori*, pickled ginger and sesame seeds.

Serves 4
Preparation time: **15 mins**

Steamed Salmon Rice with Mushrooms
(Japan)

6 dried shiitake or
Chinese mushrooms
2 cups (500 ml) boiling
water
2 cups uncooked
Japanese rice
2 tablespoons soy sauce
3 tablespoons sake
3 teaspoons rice vinegar
$^1/_2$ teaspoon salt
1 leek, white part only,
very thinly sliced (about
$^1/_2$ cup), soaked in
water
8 oz (220 g) fresh salmon
fillets, cleaned and
skin removed
4 teaspoons *mirin*
2 *shiso* (or basil) leaves,
chopped
1 sheet *nori*, lightly toasted and cut in thin
strips, to garnish (see
page 6)
1 tablespoon toasted
sesame seeds, to gar-
nish

1 Place the mushrooms into a bowl with the boiling water and soak for 10 minutes. Drain, reserving the soaking liquid, then squeeze the mushrooms gently to remove any excess liquid. Remove and discard the stems and slice the caps thinly.

2 Wash the rice and place in a rice cooker or large saucepan with the soy sauce, sake, rice vinegar, salt and 2 cups (500 ml) of the reserved mushroom soaking liquid (add cold water if needed to make 2 cups). Stir to combine.

3 Place the leek, salmon and mushrooms on top of the rice and cook according to the manufacturer's instructions. If not using a rice cooker, use a saucepan with a tight fitting lid. Bring to the boil, reduce heat to low and simmer covered until the rice is cooked, 20–25 minutes. The rice is cooked when small steam holes are visible on its surface.

4 Remove the lid, sprinkle with *mirin* and gently flake the salmon with a fork. Add the *shiso* leaves and stir lightly to combine.

6 Serve hot, topped with *nori* and sesame seeds.

Serves 4
Preparation time: 15 mins
Cooking time: 25 mins

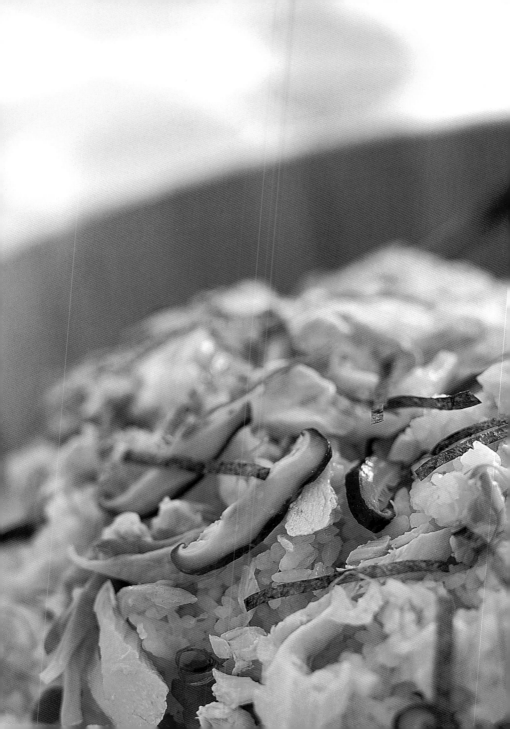

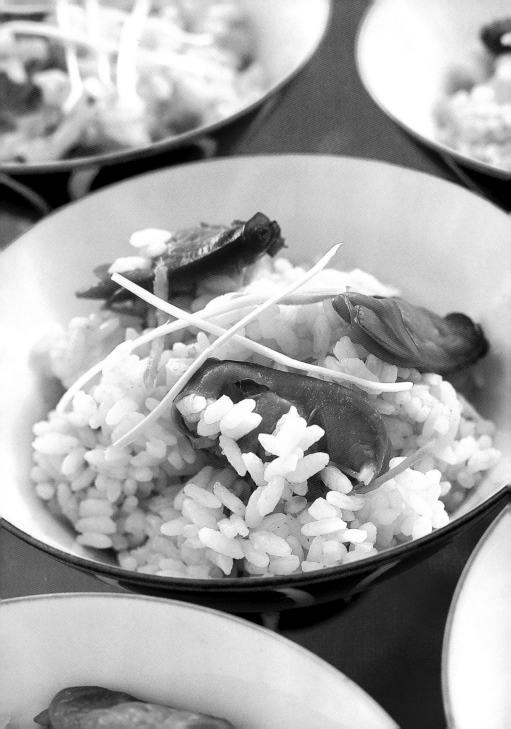

Steamed Rice with Clams (Japan)

2 lbs (1 kg) medium clams in the shell or 8 oz (220 g) fresh or canned clam meat
4 teaspoons sake
3 tablespoons soy sauce
2 teaspoons *mirin*
1/2 tablespoon finely grated fresh young ginger
6 cups freshly cooked Japanese rice
1 scallion, white part only, sliced in thin strips

Serves 4–5
Preparation time: 30 mins
Cooking time: 10 mins

1 Scrub the clams with a brush and soak in a large bowl of cold water for 5 minutes. (If using clam meat, rinse in cold water, drain and set aside). Drain and rinse well.

2 Cook the clams covered in a medium saucepan over high heat until the shells open slightly, 3–4 minutes. Add a tablespoon of water if there is not enough liquid from the clams to form some steam. Discard any clams that do not open. Drain, and when cool enough to handle, remove the clam meat and discard the shells.

3 Return clam meat to the saucepan, add the sake and cook over high heat, stirring quickly until the meat is just cooked, about 1 minute.

4 Add the soy sauce, *mirin* and ginger to the clams and continue to cook over medium heat for 1 minute. Add the clam mixture to the warm rice and gently fold through until combined. Serve immediately topped with the sliced scallions.

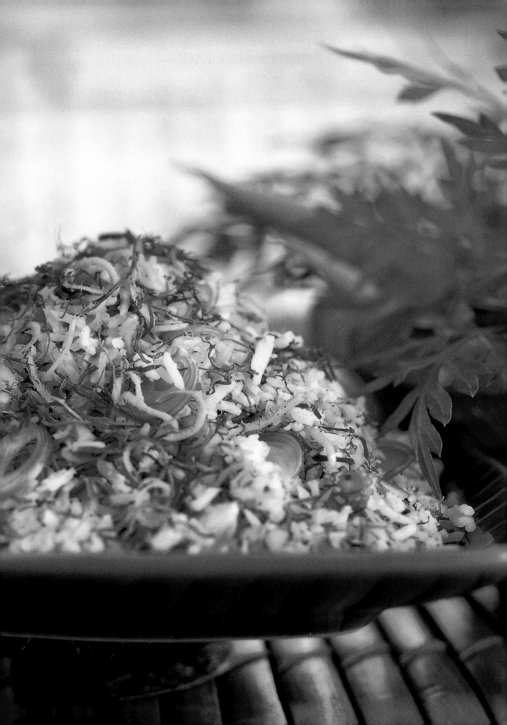

Mixed Herb Rice (Malaysia)

1 cup (110 g) grated fresh coconut
Oil for deep-frying
$^2/_3$ cup (60 g) whole dried anchovies or whitebait (*ikan bilis*) (optional)
2 tablespoons oil
3 cups cold cooked rice, separated with a fork
1 cup finely chopped mixed herbs (see note)
1 stem lemongrass, inner part of thick stem only, thinly sliced
1 torch ginger bud, thinly sliced (optional)
10 shallots, thinly sliced
1 tablespoon finely grated fresh young ginger
2 teaspoons finely grated fresh galangal
2 teaspoons finely grated fresh turmeric or $^1/_2$ teaspoon turmeric powder
$^1/_2$ teaspoon salt
$^1/_2$ teaspoon freshly ground black pepper

Serves 4
Preparation time: 25 mins
Cooking time: 30 mins

1 Dry-fry the grated coconut in a wok over very low heat, stirring constantly to prevent burning, until golden brown, about 20 minutes for fresh coconut. Cool slightly. Pound with a mortar and pestle, or process in a food processor until it is the texture of fine breadcrumbs.

2 Rinse the anchovies under running water to remove excess salt, then dry with paper towels. Heat the 2 tablespoons of oil in a small frying pan and fry the anchovies over low heat until lightly colored on both sides, about 2 minutes. Cool and shred the fish finely.

3 Combine the rice with the rest of the ingredients in a large bowl, mixing with two wooden spoons or clean hands. Serve as soon as possible after mixing.

Bunches of **mixed herbs** *(daun ulam) especially for this dish are sold in Malay market stalls and include long-stemmed mint (daun kesum or daun laksa), Asian pennywort (daun pegaga), aromatic ginger leaf (daun cekur), common mint (daun pudina), kaffir lime leaf (daun limau purut), young cashew leaves (daun cajus) and wild pepper leaf (daun kaduk). Any mixture of fragrant Asian herbs can be used, but at least 3 or 4 different herbs are needed to achieve the desired complex aromas. Thai basil, mint, polygonum, lime leaves and wild pepper leaves are traditional, but dill, celery leaf, shiso leaf and cilantro leaf can also be used. To shred the herbs, wash and pat dry with a clean cloth. Roll up a wad of herbs using the larger leaves on the outside and slice very finely using a very sharp knife.*

Torch ginger buds *also known as bunga kantan or bunga siantan, are the edible pink buds of a wild ginger plant. It is eaten raw with a dip, added to salads or used in soups and curries. They are not widely available outside of Asia and may be substituted with a tablespoon of finely sliced Vietnamese mint.*

Vegetable Biryani (India)

1 cup (150 g) peeled split mung beans
2 tablespoons ghee or oil
1 cinnamon stick, broken in half
6 cardamom pods
6 whole cloves
3 bay leaves
2 medium onions, finely chopped
2 tablespoons freshly grated ginger
1 red chili, thinly sliced
2 1/4 cups (500 g) uncooked long grain rice, washed
and drained
1 teaspoon curry powder
1 cup (160 g) fresh or frozen green peas or diced
mixed vegetables
4 cups (1 liter) water
1 1/2 teaspoons salt

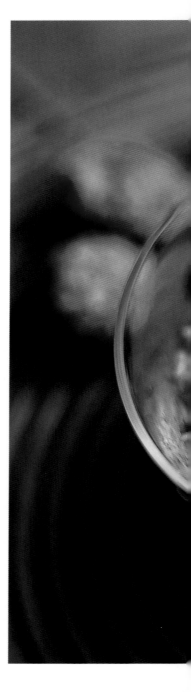

1 Dry-roast the mung beans in a wok over medium
heat until aromatic and golden brown, 3–5 minutes.
Cool thoroughly, then wash well, drain and set aside.
2 Heat the ghee or oil and fry the cinnamon, cardamom pods, cloves and bay leaves over medium
heat until aromatic, 1–2 minutes.
3 Add the onions, ginger and red chili. Stir-fry until
the onions are lightly browned, 2–3 minutes.
4 Transfer to a rice cooker. Add the rest of the ingredients and mix well, then turn on the rice cooker. If not
using a rice cooker, bring the water to the boil in a
deep pot, add all the ingredients and mix well. Reduce
the heat to very low, cover the pot and simmer gently,
stirring occasionally until rice is cooked and water,
evaporated, 20–25 minutes.
5 When rice is cooked, fluff up rice with a wooden
spoon. Serve with a salad or vegetable.

Serves 4
Preparation time: **20 mins**
Cooking time: **20 mins**

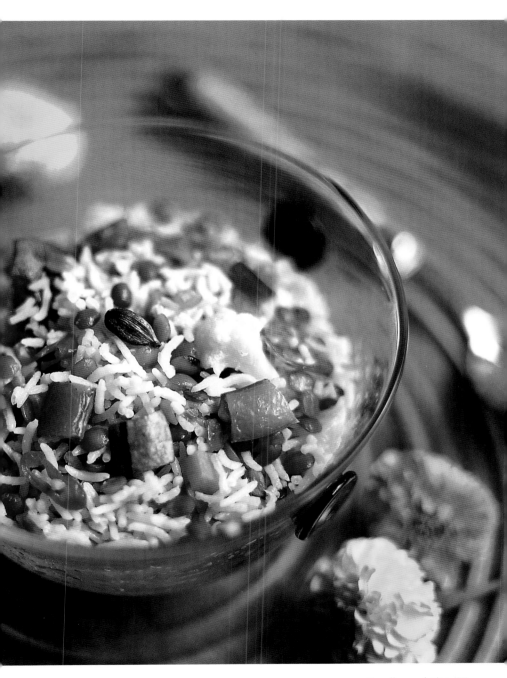

Millet and Brown Rice Congee (China)

Millet is the oldest grain on record as a staple cereal crop in China. Although it is rarely consumed any more in the West, millet remains one of the most beneficial of all grains for human health. It is also very easy to digest and it's the only grain that alkalizes rather than acidifies the stomach. Millet lends itself best to the preparation of congee and in this recipe it is combined with the hearty flavor and chewy texture of brown rice.

1 cup (200 g) uncooked brown rice
16 cups (4 liters) water
$1/2$ cup (125 g) uncooked millet
1 teaspoon salt

Seasonings
1 teaspoon sesame oil
$1/2$ teaspoon freshly ground black pepper
$1/2$ teaspoon salt
1 scallion, chopped

Serves 4
Preparation time: 5 mins
 + 3–5 hours soaking
Cooking time: $1^1/_4$ hours

1 Wash and rinse the brown rice well, then place in a large pot and add the water. Set aside to soak for 3–5 hours, or overnight.

2 Bring the water and rice to the boil, then add the millet and the salt. When water returns to a full boil, reduce the heat to medium-low, cover partially with lid to allow steam to escape and simmer until it reaches the consistency of porridge, about $1^1/_4$ hours. Stir occasionally to prevent sticking and add water as needed if it gets too dry.

3 Turn off the heat and leave covered until ready to serve.

4 Divide the Seasonings among individual serving bowls, spoon the congee on top and stir to blend the flavors.

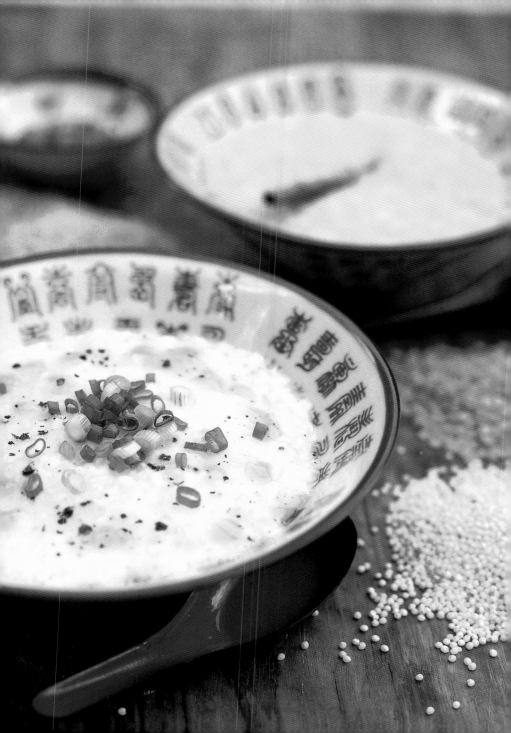

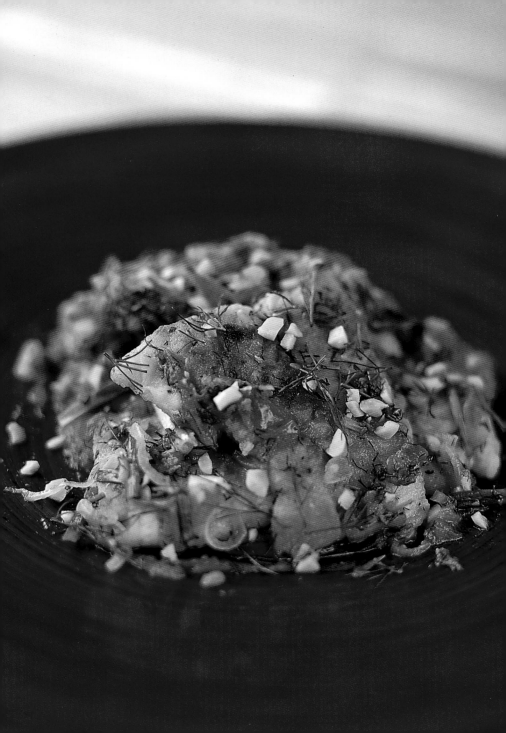

Sautéed Fish with Dill (Vietnam)

This Vietnamese fried fish sings with complementary flavors and textures, and rates high marks. This recipe will serve four as part of a larger meal, but two can finish it without any problems.

1 lb (450 g) firm-fleshed fish fillets or fish steaks
1 tablespoon fish sauce
$1/_2$ teaspoon freshly ground black pepper
2 tablespoons plain flour for dredging
4 tablespoons oil

Gravy
3 shallots, peeled and thinly sliced
1 tablespoon finely chopped garlic
3 tomatoes, cored, seeded and diced
$1^1/_2$ tablespoons fish sauce
1 teaspoon sugar
$1/_2$ cup (125 ml) cold water or chicken stock (made from chicken bouillon cubes)
2 scallions, cut into small pieces
$1/_4$ cup chopped fresh dill
2 tablespoons chopped fresh cilantro (coriander leaves)
$1/_4$ cup (50 g) coarsely chopped unsalted roasted peanuts

1 Place the fish fillets or fish steak in a large baking dish and sprinkle with the fish sauce and black pepper. Dredge the fish in the flour, shaking off excess.
2 Heat the oil in a large frying pan over medium heat and cook the fish until browned, about 2 minutes on each side. Remove the fish and set aside.
3 Drain the oil, leaving about 2 tablespoons of oil in the pan. To make the Gravy, heat the oil, then add the shallots and garlic and stir-fry for 2 minutes. Add the tomatoes and cook 2 minutes more. Add the fish sauce, sugar and water and cook, stirring occasionally, for about 5 minutes.
4 Add the scallions, dill and fresh cilantro, stirring to combine. Return the fish to the pan and stir to cover with the sauce and heat through. Place on a serving platter and serve sprinkled with the chopped peanuts.

Serves 4
Preparation time: **20 mins**
Cooking time: **10 mins**

Red-braised Fish Steak (China)

Red-braising is a traditional Chinese method of cooking meat, poultry and seafood. After searing the item to be cooked in hot oil, a fragrant sauce containing some sugar and soy sauce is poured over it, then the pan is covered and the food allowed to braise for a while. The characteristic dark red sheen is produced by the fusion of soy sauce, sugar and fat. Red braising is an excellent way to cook deep-water fish steaks or fillets.

1 1/2 lbs (675 g) fresh fish steaks or fillets (tuna, halibut, seabass, swordfish or any other firm-fleshed, deep-water fish), cut about 3/4 in (1 1/2 cm) thick
1 teaspoon salt
1/4 teaspoon pepper
6 scallions, cut into short lengths

Sauce
2 tablespoons soy sauce
2 tablespoons rice wine
1 teaspoon sugar
1 teaspoon sesame oil
1/2 teaspoon vinegar
1 tablespoon freshly grated ginger

Serves 4
Preparation time: **15 mins**
Cooking time: **10 mins**

1 Combine the Sauce ingredients and set aside.
2 Rinse the fish and pat dry with paper towels, then sprinkle both sides with salt and pepper.
3 Heat a skillet or shallow wok over medium heat and rub the entire inside surface with a piece of fresh ginger (this helps prevent sticking). Add the oil.
4 When the oil is hot, place the steaks or fillets in the pan and fry for 2 minutes on each side. Gently shake the pan to help prevent sticking.
5 Pour the Sauce over the fish. Gently shake the pan to blend and distribute the sauce evenly, then braise without a lid for 1–2 minutes.
6 Turn the fish, toss in the scallions and shake the pan. Braise for 2 more minutes and transfer to a serving dish.

For a spicier meal, add 1 tablespoon of chili paste to the sauce, or dust the cooked fish lightly with ground Sichuan pepper. If desired, garnish with freshly chopped cilantro (coriander leaves), which goes very well with most seafood dishes.

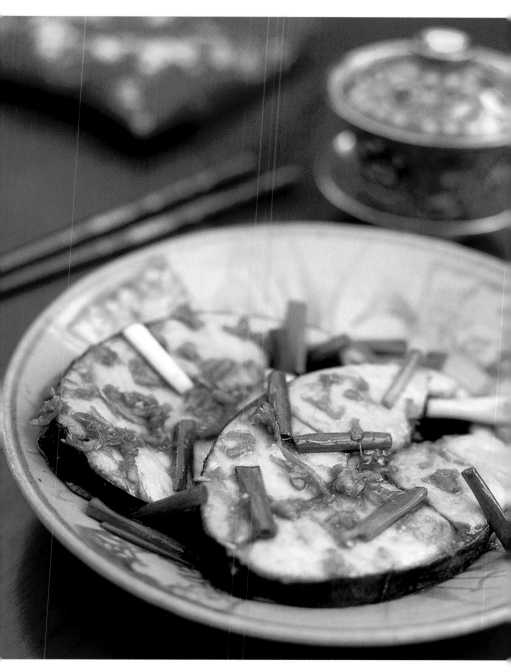

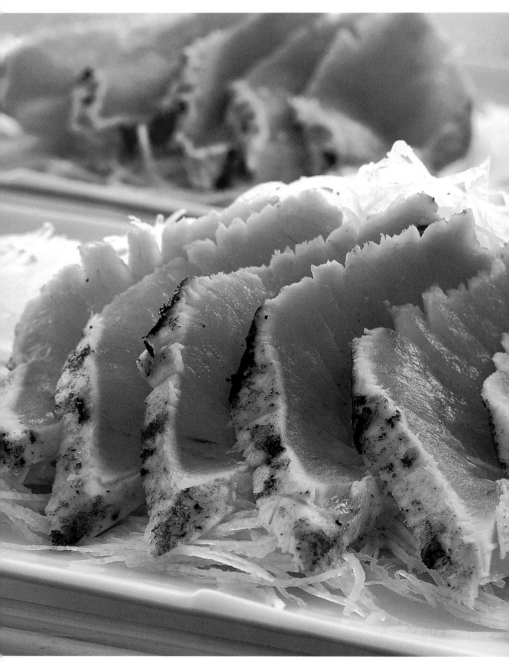

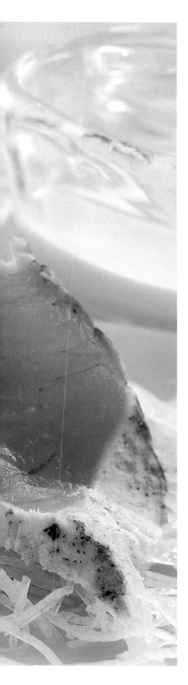

Pepper-seared Tuna (Japan)

1 lb (450 g) fresh, sashimi-quality tuna
4 teaspoons sake
4 teaspoons *mirin*
1 teaspoon *sansho* pepper or cracked black pepper
1 tablespoon oil
1 medium daikon, shredded (3–4 cups), to serve

Wasabi Dipping Sauce
$^1/_4$ cup (60 ml) high-quality mayonnaise
2–3 teaspoons *wasabi* powder or paste
2 teaspoons *mirin*
2 teaspoons sake

1 Cut the tuna into fillets that are approximately 1 in ($2^1/_2$ cm) thick and 2 in (5 cm) wide. Combine the sake and *mirin*, add the tuna and marinate for at least 30 minutes or overnight.
2 Combine the Wasabi Dipping Sauce ingredients in a bowl and set aside.
3 Drain the marinated tuna. Combine the pepper and oil in a small baking tray and roll the drained tuna in the mixture until evenly coated.
4 Heat a medium frying pan over high heat, then add the tuna and sear until all surfaces are sealed and tuna is lightly browned, about 1 minute on each side. Remove the tuna from the pan and set aside to cool. Slice the tuna on an angle into $^1/_2$-in (1-cm) thick slices and arrange overlapping on serving plates on a bed of daikon. Serve with the Wasabi Dipping Sauce.

Serves 4
Preparation time: **5 mins + 30 mins marinating**
Cooking time: **8 mins**

Chicken Steamed with Black Mushrooms
(Malaysia)

1 whole chicken (3 lbs/ 1¹/₄ kg) or 2 lbs (900 g) chicken pieces (breasts, thighs and drumsticks), fat discarded, cut into bite-sized pieces
8 dried black Chinese mushrooms, soaked in hot water, stems discarded
2 tablespoons finely diced ginger
1 tablespoon water
2 tablespoons rice wine
1 tablespoon soy sauce
1 tablespoon oyster sauce
1 teaspoon sesame oil
2 teaspoons sugar
1 teaspoon salt
¹/₂ teaspoon freshly ground white pepper
1 scallion, finely chopped

1 Put the chicken and mushrooms in a heat-proof bowl with a lid.

2 Process the ginger and water in a spice grinder, or pound ginger in a mortar, then mix with water. Put the ginger and any liquid in a small sieve and press down with the back of a spoon to extract the ginger juice. Sprinkle the ginger juice, rice wine, soy and oyster sauces, sesame oil, sugar, salt and pepper over the chicken and mushrooms, massaging with your hand to mix well. Cover the bowl and refrigerate 1 hour.

3 When ready to cook, put the bowl inside a steamer filled with water, or place on a rack set in a deep saucepan half-filled with water. Cover the steamer or pan and steam over medium heat until the chicken is cooked, 30–40 minutes, adding a little more boiling water to the steamer every 10 minutes. Transfer to a serving dish, sprinkle with the scallions and serve hot with plain rice.

Serves 4–6
Preparation time: 15 mins + 1 hour marinating time
Cooking time: 30–40 mins

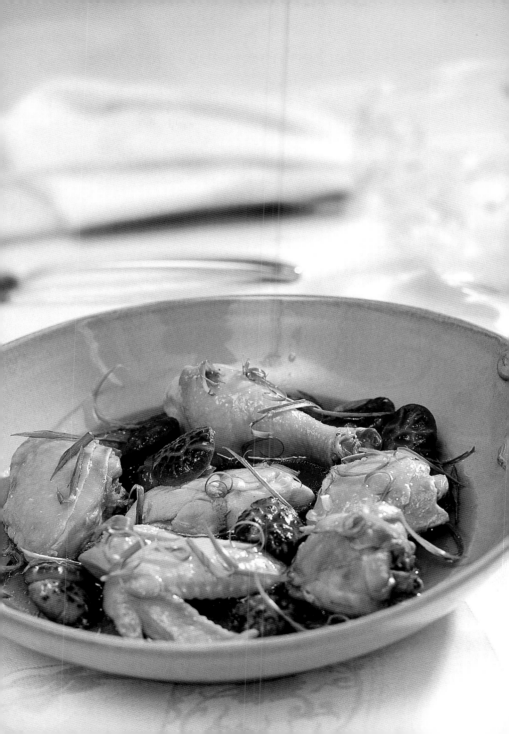

Braised Chicken and Lotus Root (Japan)

8 dried shiitake or
Chinese mushrooms
soaked in hot water
1 small lotus root (about
5 oz/140 g), peeled
2 tablespoons rice
wine vinegar
1 medium carrot, peeled
1 tablespoon oil
10 oz (300 g) boneless
chicken meat, cubed
3 tablespoons sake
1$^1/_2$ teaspoons dashi
powder dissolved in
1$^1/_4$ cups (300 ml)
water
2 tablespoons *mirin*
2–3 tablespoons soy
sauce
12 snow peas, tops and
tails removed

Serves 4
Preparation time: 20 mins
Cooking time: 35 mins

1 Drain the mushrooms, squeezing each mushroom gently to remove excess liquid. Reserve the soaking liquid. Remove and discard the mushroom stems and cut the caps in half.

2 Cut the lotus root in half widthwise and then into $^1/_4$ in ($^1/_2$ cm) slices. Place in a small bowl with the vinegar and enough water to cover. Let soak for 10 minutes, then drain.

3 Cut the carrot into rounds on an angle, rolling a quarter turn each cut.

4 Heat the oil in a medium saucepan over high heat. Add the chicken, skin side down, and cook until golden brown, 1–2 minutes each side. Carefully drain and discard the excess oil from the pan.

5 Add the mushrooms, drained lotus root, carrot and sake and stir to combine. Add the *dashi* mixture and bring to the boil, removing any impurities from the surface with a spoon or paper towel. Add the *mirin* and half of the soy sauce, and place a small saucepan lid directly on top of the vegetables to keep them from moving around too much during cooking. Cover the pan and boil for 5 minutes. Reduce the heat and simmer for 10 more minutes.

6 Remove the small saucepan lid, add the remaining soy sauce and the snow peas and continue to simmer covered for 5 minutes.

7 Remove from the heat and let stand for 5 minutes before serving in small bowls with a little of the cooking liquid.

Lotus roots are the edible roots of the lotus plant that look a bit like sweet potatoes that are linked like sausages. When sliced, this starchy vegetable with a crisp texture and mild flavor reveals a lace-like pattern of holes. They are available both fresh and in packages of dried slices in Asian food shops.

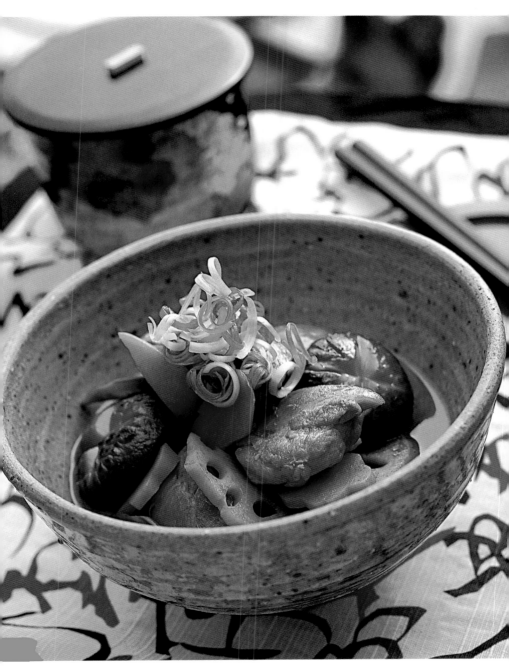

Exotic Flavored Chicken (China)

The term "exotic flavor" (*guai wei*) refers to a potent combination of spices and seasonings that combines the full spectrum of taste sensations in one harmonious blend. In addition, this blend of herbs provides a stimulating therapeutic boost to the whole system. To prepare this dish, you must first poach a whole chicken the Chinese way. This step takes about $1^1/_2$ hours (but virtually no effort) and may be done well in advance, even the day before.

1 whole chicken (about 3 lbs/$1^1/_2$ kg)
1 cup (250 ml) rice wine
4 scallions, coarsely chopped, 2 tablespoons reserved to garnish
6 slices ginger
1 head iceberg lettuce
2 tablespoons chopped cilantro (coriander leaves) or parsley to garnish

Sauce
2 tablespoons finely chopped garlic
2 tablespoons finely chopped ginger
4 scallions, finely sliced
1 teaspoon ground Sichuan pepper
1 teaspoon salt
1 teaspoon sugar
1 tablespoon sesame oil
1 tablespoon olive oil
$^1/_2$ teaspoon vinegar
2 tablespoons soy sauce
1 tablespoon chili sauce
1 tablespoon sesame paste (or tahini) mixed with 2 tablespoons hot water

1 To poach the chicken, fill a large pot two-thirds full with water, then add the wine, scallions and ginger slices. Bring the water to a rapid boil, then add the whole chicken, breast-side down. When the water returns to the boil, cover the pot tightly, reduce the heat to low and simmer for 5 minutes. Turn off the heat, wrap the pot well in several towels to keep it hot, then set the chicken aside to poach itself for about $1^1/_2$ hours.
2 When the chicken is done, remove it from the water and set it on a rack to drain until ready to use (refrigerate if using the following day).
3 To prepare the Sauce, place garlic, ginger and scallions in a heatproof bowl. Add the ground Sichuan pepper, salt and sugar. Heat the sesame and olive oils in a small skillet or wok until smoking hot, then pour over the spices in the bowl and let it sizzle. Add the vinegar, soy sauce, chili sauce and sesame paste, one at a time, stirring each well into the Sauce.
4 Cut the chicken into parts (legs, wings, breast, etc.), then either chop them into bite-sized pieces with a heavy cleaver, or pull the meat from the bones with your fingers.
5 Finely slice the lettuce and arrange it on a serving platter, arrange the chicken meat neatly on top, then pour or spoon the sauce evenly over the chicken. Serve garnished with fresh cilantro or parsley.

Serves 4–6
Preparation time: **2 hours**
Assembling time: **15 mins**

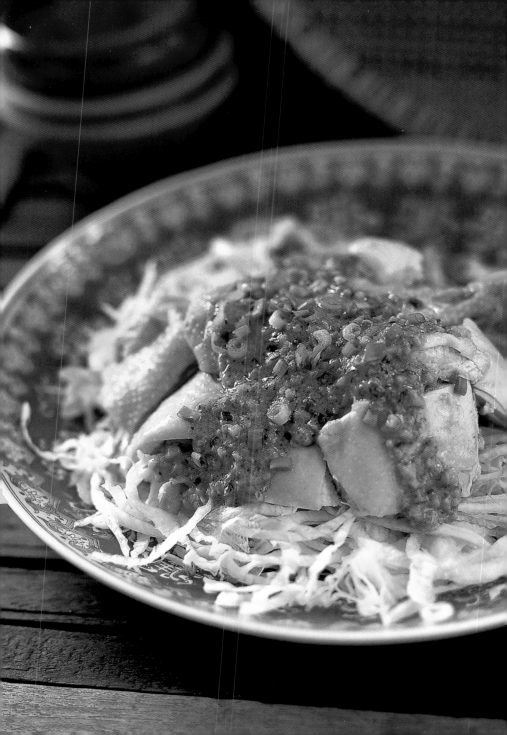

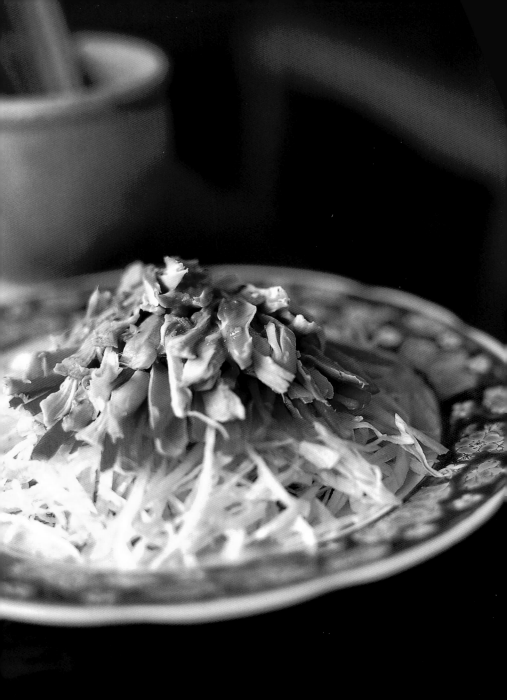

Shredded Chicken with Sesame Sauce
(China)

Often referred to in the English versions of Chinese menus as Bon Bon Chicken, presumably because it's pronounced *bang bang ji* in Chinese, this is one of the most popular chicken concoctions in Sichuan. The term *bang bang* is equivalent to the English word drumstick as a vernacular reference to the leg of the chicken. This dish is usually served as a cold appetizer at the beginning of a meal, but it may also be the main event in a simple lunch.

1 lb (450 g) chicken legs
$1/2$ head iceberg or other lettuce, finely shredded
1 red bell pepper (capsicum), cut in thin strips
$1/2$ teaspoon sea salt
1 teaspoon sesame oil

Sauce
$2^1/2$ tablespoons dark Chinese sesame paste or tahini
$1/4$ cup (60 ml) chicken stock (made from chicken bouillon cubes) or water
$1/2$ teaspoon ground Sichuan pepper
2 teaspoons sugar
1 teaspoon vinegar
1 teaspoon red chili oil
2 teaspoons sesame oil
2 teaspoons thick soy sauce
$1/2$ teaspoon salt
1 tablespoon freshly grated ginger
1 tablespoon finely chopped garlic

Serves 2–4
Preparation time: **20 mins**
Cooking time: **1 hour**

1 Poach the chicken legs by placing them in a large pot with sufficient water to cover them by $1^1/4$ in (3 cm) and bring to the boil. Reduce the heat, cover tightly, then simmer for 10 minutes. Turn off the heat and set aside to poach in hot water for 30 minutes. Remove the chicken from the water and drain.
2 Spread the lettuce evenly on a serving plate. Place the bell pepper strips into a bowl with the salt and mix with your fingers to soften them. Add the sesame oil and continue to mix with your fingers until well coated, then arrange the strips evenly over the shredded lettuce.
3 Mix the Sauce by blending the sesame paste or tahini with the chicken stock or water in a bowl. Add the ground Sichuan pepper and mix well, then add the remaining ingredients, one at a time, stirring continuously with a fork until well mixed.
4 Remove the skin from the poached chicken and pull the meat from the bones. Tear the meat into fine shreds and pile the shredded chicken on top of the lettuce and bell peppers. Drizzle the sauce evenly over the chicken and serve.

This dish may be garnished with chopped fresh cilantro (coriander leaves) or chopped scallions. You may also use other parts of the chicken, particularly if you wish to prepare a larger portion. For example, you may poach and shred a whole chicken. To poach a whole chicken, follow the instructions for Exotic Flavored Chicken on page 88.

Hainanese Chicken Rice (Singapore)

1 teaspoon rice wine
2 tablespoons light soy sauce
1 chicken, (about 3 lbs/ 1¹/₂ kg)
2 slices fresh ginger
1 clove garlic, bruised
1 scallion, chopped
Water for boiling chicken
1 teaspoon sesame oil
¹/₂ teaspoon salt
1 small cucumber, seeds removed and cut into thin strips, to garnish
Soy sauce, to serve

Rice
2 cups (400 g) uncooked long grain rice
4 cups (1 liter) chicken stock (from simmering chicken)

Chili Ginger Sauce
2–4 large red chilies
6 cloves garlic
2 slices fresh ginger
2 teaspoons chicken stock (from simmering chicken)
¹/₄ teaspoon salt

Serves 4–6
Preparation time: 20 mins
Cooking time:
  1 hour 10 mins

1 Mix the rice wine and 2 teaspoons of the soy sauce and rub the mixture inside the chicken. Put the ginger, garlic and scallions inside the chicken.

2 Select a pot just large enough to hold the chicken and add sufficient water to cover the chicken. Bring the water to the boil, then put in the chicken, cover the pan and turn off heat immediately. Leave the chicken for 5 minutes, then lift the chicken, drain the water and lower the chicken back into the water. Cover the pot, but do not reheat. Set the chicken aside to poach for another 25 minutes.

3 Drain the chicken again and put it back in the water. Turn the heat on, bring the water almost to the boil, then turn the heat off and let the chicken stand for 30 minutes. By this time, it should be cooked; leave the chicken in the water until ready to serve.

4 While the chicken is cooking, prepare the Chili Ginger Sauce by grinding all ingredients in a spice grinder or blender until finely ground and well blended. Set aside.

5 To prepare the Rice put the rice in a pot with enough stock to cover it by about 1 in (2¹/₂ cm). Bring quickly to the boil, lower the heat and simmer with the pan half covered until the water is entirely absorbed. Reduce the heat to low, cover the pan and cook another 10 minutes, until all the liquid is absorbed. Fluff up the rice with a fork and remove from the heat.

6 Combine the remaining soy sauce with the sesame oil and salt. Drain the chicken, then rub the soy mixture on the outside. Chop the chicken into bite-sized pieces with a cleaver. Place chicken on a serving dish garnished with cucumber slices. Serve with soy sauce and Chili Ginger Sauce.

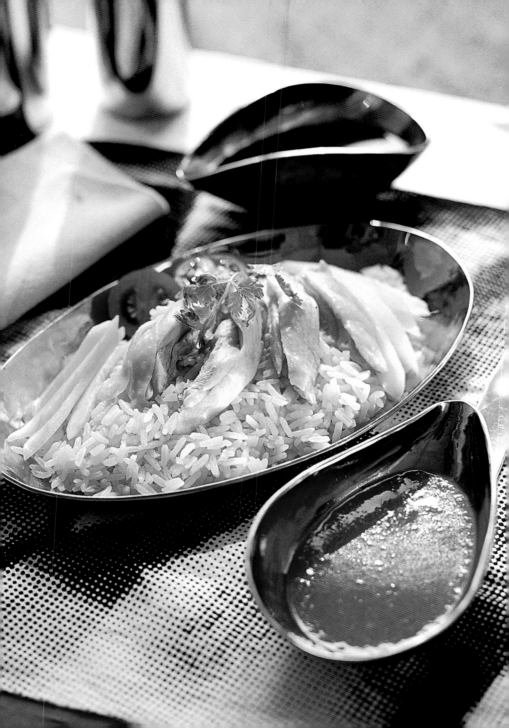

Beef and White Leek with Sweet Soy Dressing (Japan)

8 oz (225 g) beef sirloin or fillet steak, thinly sliced
1 tablespoon oil
2 teaspoons sake
2 teaspoons soy sauce
1 leek, white part only, sliced in very thin strips lengthwise (about $1/4$ cup), soaked in water, to garnish
1 teaspoon sesame seeds, roasted, to garnish

Sweet Soy Dressing
2 tablespoons rice wine vinegar
4 teaspoons soy sauce,
4 teaspoons *mirin*
2 tablespoons sake
2 teaspoons sugar

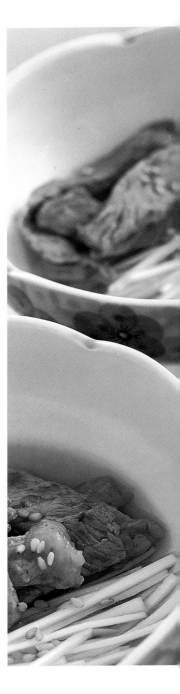

1 Place the beef in a medium bowl with the oil, sake
and soy sauce and toss to combine. Set aside to
marinate while making the Sweet Soy Dressing
2 To make the Sweet Soy Dressing, combine all the
ingredients in a small pan. Heat rapidly over high
heat, stirring until the sugar dissolves. Remove from
the heat and set aside.
3 Heat a medium non-stick frying pan over high heat
and cook half of the sliced beef until just cooked, 1–2
minutes on each side. Repeat with remaining beef
slices.
4 Divide the meat between 4 shallow bowls, pour
over the hot Sweet Soy Dressing and let stand for 5
minutes. Serve warm or cold garnished with drained
sliced leek and roasted sesame seeds.

Serves 4
Preparation time: **15 mins**
Cooking time: **10 mins**

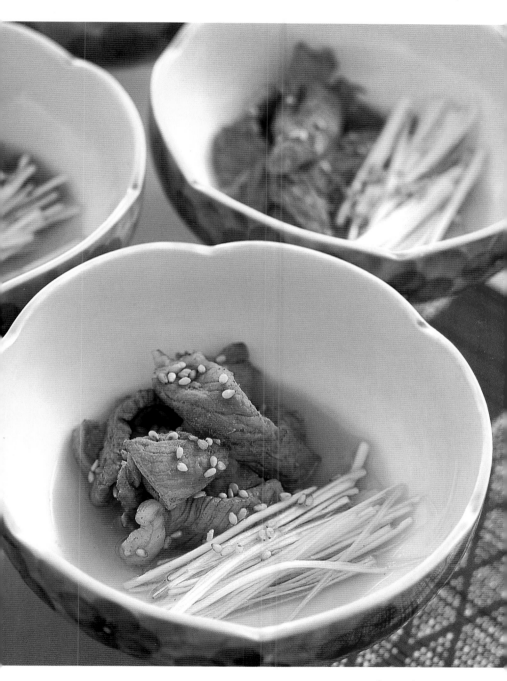

Complete Recipe Listing